OXFORD MEDICAL PUBLICATIONS

Medical Audit in Primary Health Care

D0300149

OXFORD GENERAL PRACTICE SERIES

Editorial Board

Medical Audit in Primary Health Care

Oxford General Practice Series • 25

Edited by

MARTIN LAWRENCE
General Practitioner,
Chipping Norton, Oxfordshire

and

THEO SCHOFIELD
General Practitioner,
Shipston-on-Stour, Warwickshire

OXFORD   NEW YORK   TOKYO
OXFORD UNIVERSITY PRESS
1993

Oxford University Press, Walton Street, Oxford OX2 6DP

Oxford   New York   Toronto
Delhi   Bombay   Calcutta   Madras   Karachi
Kuala Lumpur   Singapore   Hong Kong   Tokyo
Nairobi   Dar es Salaam   Cape Town
Melbourne   Auckland   Madrid
and associated companies in
Berlin   Ibadan

Oxford is a trade mark of Oxford University Press

Published in the United States
by Oxford University Press Inc., New York

© Martin Lawrence and Theo Schofield, 1993

A catalogue record for this book is available from the British Library

Library of Congress Cataloging in Publication Data
(Data applied for)

ISBN 0–19–262267–6 (pbk)

Set by Advance Typesetting Ltd, Oxfordshire
Printed in Great Britain by
Biddles Ltd, Guildford & King's Lynn

Ever tried. Ever failed.
No matter.
Try again. Fail again. Fail better.

Samuel Beckett

The audit cycle

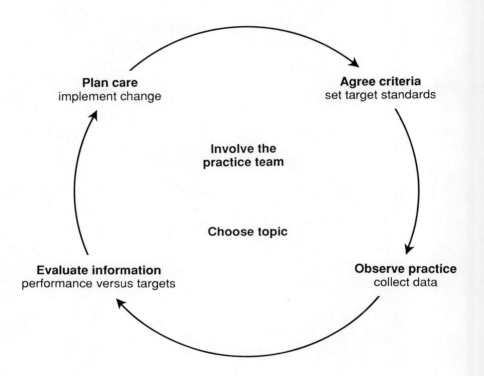

Plan care
implement change

Agree criteria
set target standards

Involve the practice team

Choose topic

Evaluate information
performance versus targets

Observe practice
collect data

Contents

Contributors

Angela Coulter BA, M.Sc. Deputy Director, Health Services Research Unit, University Department of Public Health and Primary Care, Gibson Building, Radcliffe Infirmary, Oxford

Andrew Farmer MA, MRCGP General Practitioner, The Health Centre, East Street, Thame, Oxon

Ray Fitzpatrick MA, M.Sc., Ph.D. University Lecturer in Medical Sociology, University Department of Public Health and Primary Care, Gibson Building, Radcliffe Infirmary, Oxford

Alan Forbes MRCP General Practitioner and Chairman (1990–2) of Liverpool MAAG Princes Park Health Centre, Bentley Road, Liverpool

George Freeman MA, MRCP, FRCGP General Practitioner and Senior Lecturer in Primary Medical Care, Aldermoor Health Centre, Aldermoor Close, Southampton

John Hasler OBE, MD, FRCGP General Practitioner and Regional Adviser in General Practice, Oxford Regional Committee for Postgraduate Medical Education and Training, Medical School Offices, John Radcliffe Hospital, Oxford

Peter Havelock FRCGP General Practitioner and Chairman of Buckinghamshire MAAG, The Pound House Surgery, 8 The Green, Wooburn Green, Bucks

Neil Johnson MA, MRCP, MRCGP General Practitioner, The Medical Centre, Badgers Crescent, Shipston-on-Stour, Warwickshire

Martin Lawrence MA, MRCP, FRCGP General Practitioner and Chairman of Oxfordshire MAAG, West Street Surgery, Chipping Norton, Oxon, and Lecturer in General Practice, University Department of Public Heath and Primary Care, Gibson Building, Radcliffe Infirmary, Oxford

David Mant MA, M.Sc., MRCGP, MFPHM General Practitioner and Lecturer in General Practice, ICRF General Practice Research Unit, University Department of Public Health and Primary Care, Gibson Building, Radcliffe Infirmary, Oxford

David Metcalfe OBE, FRCGP, FFPHM General Practitioner and Professor of General Practice, Rusholme Health Centre, Walmer Street, Manchester

Karen Munro B.Sc., SRD, Dip.HE Primary Care Development Consultant, 3 Riddings Road, Hale, Altrincham, Cheshire

Thomas O'Dowd MD, FRCGP General Practitioner and Senior Lecturer in General Practice, Department of General Practice, University of Nottingham Medical School, Queen's Medical Centre, Nottingham

Mary Pierce MA, M.Sc., MRCGP General Practitioner and Lecturer in General Practice, Guy's Hospital, 15 St Thomas Street, London

Philip Reilly MD, FRCGP, MICGP General Practitioner and Professor of General Practice, Department of General Practice, Queen's University of Belfast, Dunluce Health Centre, Belfast

Theo Schofield MA, MRCP, FRCGP General Practitioner, The Medical Centre, Badgers Crescent, Shipston-on-Stour, Warwickshire, and Lecturer in General Practice, University Department of Public Health and Primary Care, Gibson Building, Radcliffe Infirmary, Oxford

Patricia Yudkin MA Statistician, ICRF General Practice Research Unit, University Department of Public Health and Primary Care, Gibson Building, Radcliffe Infirmary, Oxford

Introduction

Medical audit is sweeping through primary care like a gale—there is an overwhelming momentum, but it is not always clear where it has developed from, what it really is, or where it is going. Havoc can be wreaked especially on the unprepared, but there is great potential to harness the energy and make it productive.

The forces which have combined to develop this momentum are several.

1. There has been a dramatic improvement in records in medical care. We have moved from Lloyd George envelopes, through the introduction of record cards, to computerization, in less than 20 years. Huge quantities of data are available, evaluating rather than collecting it has become the challenge.
2. General practice vocational training developed greatly in the 1980s, with compulsory training being introduced in 1981. There is now a cohort of young, well-trained doctors ready and keen to take on this evaluation.
3. Practice teams, supported by the changes of the 1966 General Practice Charter, have matured over the last decade. The educational development of practice nurses, practice managers, and other clerical staff, as well as the revitalization of the health visitor's role, has stimulated an interest in the larger and potentially effective primary health care team.
4. Public awareness and political trends demand that the medical profession becomes more accountable. Quality of service and of care is now questioned and expected, and is no longer the prerogative of the profession to determine.

All these powerful forces are driving audit, while many in the medical profession are still unsure as to what it is and how to do it. Indeed, much perception of audit has been distorted. Early exercises in audit were seen as the interest of the minority, causing a lot of work for little benefit. More recently it has been considered an externally imposed activity, restricting freedom and producing threat—a perception reinforced by the large amount of data which has been demanded by the 1990 general practice contract. Such insistence on data collection has reinforced a further misapprehension about audit, that it necessarily involves large amounts of data collection, usually requiring computers and statistical analysis. Indeed, this emphasis on data is in danger of suggesting that data collection is the most important aspect of audit, overlooking the more crucial areas of planning change and setting targets. There has also been a tendency to undervalue the interactive areas of primary care which cannot be evaluated in a numerical way.

This book attempts to clarify many of the issues and redress the balance. It is both theoretical and practical. The underlying principles of audit are clearly and concisely expounded; its potential for service improvement, developing the education of all health professionals, and maintaining public confidence are emphasized. In this way enthusiasm and excitement for primary care can be restored in the face of increasing control and monitoring by authorities.

The book also supplies the need for practices to have detailed examples of audit in action. Thus, the energy that it is hoped will be developed by reading Parts I and II can find outlet in the practical examples given in Part III.

There is a tension between external monitoring and professional audit. If confidential audit is to satisfy the requirements of accountability then the profession must face up to its responsibilities in this area. The principles are discussed in Chapter 3 by Professor David Metcalfe, while Part IV concentrates on the role of Medical Audit Advisory Groups (MAAGs) and ways of auditing the audits themselves.

Hardly anyone whose work concerns primary health care is now not concerned with audit.

Firstly, all general practitioners are now expected to take part in audit, by the Government, by their peers, and, increasingly, by their patients. In particular, training practices will need to develop theory with trainees and also to help trainees implement their own audits.

Secondly, MAAGs and their visiting teams will need to clarify their views on audit—about which they will have to convince other doctors—and to provide a 'menu' of audits which practices might begin.

Thirdly, the other professions in primary medical care are increasingly going to be involved in audit. Practice nursing is developing, and so is the education of practice nurses; health visitors are rediscovering their role in the wider practice team; practice managers and clerical staff are increasingly taking on a role in audit, and so developing their professional stature.

Fourthly, Family Health Service Authorities (FHSAs) and their medical advisers need to be able to reconcile their responsibility for the standard of primary medical care in their districts with the profession's need for self regulation and the maintenance of standards. This book may help FHSA staff to appreciate the potentials and limits of working together with the profession.

Fifthly, hospital doctors may find the book interesting. We believe that general practice leads the field in many areas of audit. Several of the ideas in this book may be new to hospital doctors and readily transferable.

Finally, audit is developing overseas as it is in the UK. Several countries, especially Scandinavian countries and the Netherlands, have systems of medical care not dissimilar to those in the UK, and there is thus great scope for exchanging ideas and methodologies. With developing economic and political unity, all European countries will be increasingly looking to each others' systems for ideas in achieving greater economy and better quality assurance.

HOW TO READ THIS BOOK

The book is divided into four sections. Part I describes the theoretical basis of audit; Part II the method by which audit can be carried out; Part III gives examples of various audits which can be carried out in primary care; and Part IV shows how advisory groups can help practices, and how audit itself can be evaluated.

Some readers may prefer to study the theory in Parts I and II before considering the examples. Others may prefer to go directly to Part III for help in implementing an audit in practice, referring back to Parts I and II for theoretical justification and support when it is required. Readers who choose to implement first and read the theory after may choose to start on a major area of medical care (for example, Chapters 9–12 and 15) or to test the water more gradually by looking first at one of the shorter audits (for example, Chapter 14).

Part I
The basis of medical audit

1 What is medical audit?

Martin Lawrence

Audit is such an unsatisfactory term that it is hard to understand how it ever became adopted by the medical profession. Its derivation from the Latin *audio* implies listening rather than doing, passivity rather than an active endeavour to change. Its usage in the accountancy and business world implies external scrutiny of activity with the promise of corrective action, rather than a professional commitment to improvement.

Perhaps it was adopted because early examples of the audit of medical care were externally organized reviews of hospital medical care provision, heavily concerned with examining the outcome of clinical care, rather than searching for an overall improvement in medical services. For example, the confidential enquiry into maternal deaths has been a long running — and successful — assessment of the clinical outcome of pregnancy, but with little concern for patient acceptability.

In primary health care, medical audit developed a momentum only during the 1970s. Prior to 1966 facilities for general practitioners in the UK were so sparse that most doctors had little time for anything other than reactive care on a day-to-day basis. The General Practice Charter of 1966 (British Medical Association 1965) encouraged group practice, enabled the development of adequate premises, and encouraged doctors to employ more staff, with the result that general practitioners began to examine the quality of their care, rather than just react to the pressure of demand. Following the introduction of the Charter, activity and writing in the field of audit increased dramatically. Not surprisingly general practitioners adopted the word audit, already used by those reviewing care in hospitals. Many authors provided their own definitions of audit, often including the word quality. Indeed, in 1983 the project launched by the Royal College of General Practitioners was called the 'Quality Initiative', despite the fact that its major aim was clearly audit, 'to define specific objectives for patient care and monitor the extent to which those objectives are met' (Royal College of General Practitioners 1985). Nevertheless, general usage of the term audit has persisted.

Shaw (1980) demonstrated the extent of confusion about the term, under the heading 'Audit by any other name'. He listed 14 words in three columns, and pointed out that by combining any one word from each column it is possible to produce 96 phrases that had been, or could be, used to mean review of health care.

Medical	Care	Evaluation
Health	Standards	Assessment
Clinical	Activity	Assurance
Professional	Quality	Audit
		Review
		Monitoring

Shaw commented on the paradox that on the one hand all these terms are similar, and therefore we should not get too excited in battling over which one to use: and on the other hand the differences between terms, if not recognized, result in misunderstanding and disagreement. In particular, the terms in the third column represent a gradation from research (evaluation), through internal review, to external review (monitoring) — and since 'audit' is often used to cover the whole range it is hardly surprising that confusion and strife result.

In the face of differing interpretations Sheldon, in his landmark Butterworth Essay (1982), wrote that 'it is time to agree finally upon its meaning, and the meaning of numerous related phrases'. Sheldon went on to offer a definition as:

Medical audit is a study of some part of the structure, process and outcome of medical care, carried out by those personally engaged in the activity concerned, to measure whether set objectives have been attained, and thus assess the quality of care delivered.

This was very helpful at the time, but clearly cannot be accepted as a final definition, since it now needs further development. For instance, it has nothing to say about change, or improvement, or repeated review, all of which would now be regarded as essential components.

Usage determines the definition of words. We cannot avoid words that have been used before, and we cannot define them for ourselves. What we must do is attempt to come to an understanding of terms which is as precise as possible. This chapter seeks to contribute to such understanding, and the concluding glossary sets out how the terms are used in the context of this book.

AUDIT AND QUALITY

While *audit* is a word which suffers because it has no intuitive meaning, *quality* is quite otherwise. Although quality may be hard to define, we all know what we mean by it — it is something which describes the *goodness* of our care. Black (1990) has made such goodness more precise by identifying four dimensions of quality — effectiveness, equity, humanity, and efficiency — thus emphasizing not only the medical perspective concerned with clinical effectiveness, but also the views of the patients with their emphasis on care, and society with its concern for cost.

Common sense determines that, rather than attempt to define terms such as audit that we do not intuitively understand, it is easier to describe the review of performance in terms of quality—quality that we need first to assess, then to improve, and finally to assure is maintained.

Quality assessment is the process of evaluating the current level of performance; *quality improvement* involves assessment but also a process of change and improvement; *quality assurance* requires both the first two stages and then the assurance of maintained good quality, which must require repeating the process of assessment and improvement. This can be viewed as a Venn diagram of increasing circles (Fig. 1.1).

Such an interpretation of quality assurance involves only a slight adaptation of the definition advanced by Black (1990):

The assessment of the quality of medical care, the efforts to improve the provision of that care, and procedures to ensure that good quality is maintained.

It is not possible to consider all medical care at once. Implementation of quality assurance has to be taken a topic at a time, and this implementation is the process of medical audit. Using the definition of Marinker (1990), medical audit is:

The attempt to improve the quality of medical care by measuring the performance of those providing that care, by considering the performance in relation to desired standards, and by improving on this performance.

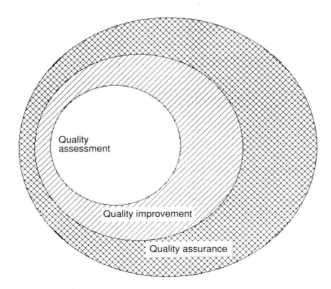

Fig. 1.1 Components of quality assurance.

Medical audit can be viewed as a cycle, of which different parts correspond to assessment and improvement of the quality of the topic being considered (Fig. 1.2). Only by competion of the cycle can the quality be assured.

One audit, even well conducted, may not give much insight into the overall quality of medical care; for that a selected range of audits need to be conducted. But if adequate topics are chosen, covering the major areas of medical care and all aspects of quality—effectiveness, efficiency, humanity, and equity—then a series of medical audits can together move towards providing quality assurance. For this reason the choosing of the topic for each audit is central to the procedure (Fig. 1.3).

The elements of the cycle are involving the team; agreeing criteria and levels of performance; observing practice and collecting data; evaluating information; planning care and implementing change; and repeating the cycle.

Involving the team

It has been suggested in the past that medical audit should refer to audit carried out amongst doctors, and that clinical audit should refer to audits carried out involving all members of medical care teams. Since primary health care teams in the UK now run an integrated system of care delivery this is not a helpful

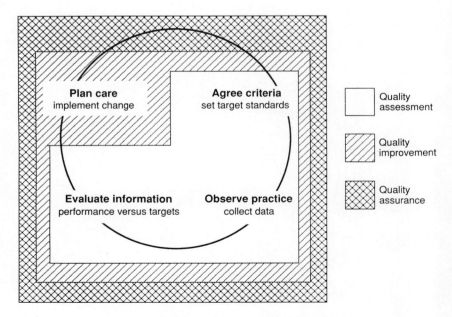

Fig. 1.2 Medical audit and quality assurance.

subdivision. Even though we may be saddled with the term 'medical audit', in primary health care it is considered to include audit carried out by any members of the primary health care team, doctors, nurses, and clerical staff.

This has major advantages both in the conduct of audit and in the commitment of the team to change, and is discussed more fully in Chapter 17.

Choosing the topic

It has already been argued that audit topics must cover a wide spectrum of medical care if medical audits are to provide quality assurance for a practice. But a start has to be made, and it is important that the start should be both interesting and manageable.

The topic chosen should be interesting, important, and amenable to change. It needs to be relevant to the practice, and audit has been shown to be less likely to be successful if the subject is imposed from outside. Availability of data is not a good reason for conducting an audit, it is more important to choose the topic and find the information on which to assess it, than to assess an activity just because data are available.

Agreeing criteria and levels of performance

To be able to interpret information or determine how successful planned changes in care have been, it is essential to describe what we are doing and define what it is that we are trying to achieve. We require precise and selective statements against which an assessment can be made.

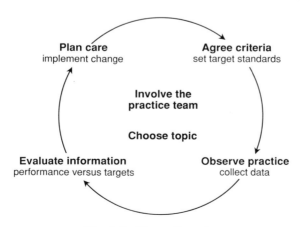

Fig. 1.3 The audit cycle.

Any topic of care or practice activity which we choose to assess consists of a large number of *elements:* so many that we must select a few for the purposes of assessment.

Our aim will be to base our assessment on those elements which are good *indicators* of care. An appropriate indicator will satisfy three conditions:

1. It will be important in determining the outcome of care or will be a desired outcome itself.
2. It will be definable or measurable.
3. It will be something which can be changed by those being assessed.

For instance, in hypertensive care, diastolic blood pressure is a good indicator because it relates to risk, its reduction is effective in reducing that risk, it can be measured, and it can be modified by treatment. In auditing access, the waiting time to be given a routine appointment is related to the humanity, effectiveness, and perhaps even the equity of care, and it can also be measured and modified.

Indicators identify the elements of care to be looked at. They do not necessarily provide satisfactory yardsticks for assessment. For this purpose, Donabedian (1982) suggests that an element needs to be defined so precisely that it is possible to say whether it is present or absent—yes or no. Elements defined so precisely can be referred to as *criteria.*

For example, in hypertension control the level of diastolic blood pressure is an indicator, but 'Is the diastolic blood pressure below 100 mmHg?', or 'Is the diastolic blood pressure below 90 mmHg?' are criteria. In assessing access, the number of days wait for an appointment is the indicator; that a patient should not have to wait more than two days is a criterion.

The advantage of defining a criterion precisely is that it is then possible to measure the extent to which that criterion is achieved, the *level of performance.*

Thus, one might find, or set, a target that 80 per cent of hypertensives on treatment have a diastolic blood pressure of less than 95 mmHg; or 90 per cent of patients could make an appointment in fewer than two days. One can then say that a *criterion* together with a *level of performance* in attaining it indicate a *standard* for that element of care (Fig. 1.4). This definition of standard is one which is increasingly being adopted. Black (1990) writes 'Standards refer to the level of compliance with a criterion'; Difford (1990) 'Criterion and performance together constitute a 'standard''; and Donabedian (1986) 'a precise, quantitative specification of the state of a criterion'. It offers a measure for Marinker's (1990) 'performance that the auditors have set themselves to achieve', or the North of England Study's (1990) 'statement of what a doctor's performance ought to be'.

The reasons for, and the implications of, defining standards in terms of criteria and levels of performance will be described more fully in Part II, Chapter 5, which describes the practical implementation of this stage of the audit cycle.

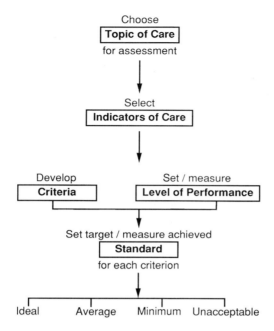

Target standards reflect *intended* quality of care.
Achieved standards reflect *delivered* quality of care.

Fig. 1.4   The definition of a standard for an element of care.

Observing practice and collecting data

'Not all that counts can be counted, and not all that can be counted counts' (Platt 1967).

The level of performance of some criteria (for example, blood pressure control) can be measured or counted, while others (for example, the exploration of patients' ideas about their problem during a consultation) can only be judged from observation or patient reports. Both are valid indicators of quality and the issue is whether the measurements or judgements can be made reliable. There is a danger of overvaluing numbers and many of the audits described later in the book depend on description and judgement.

There is also a common misapprehension that audit cannot be done without a computer and that computer data *is* audit. This has led to the overvaluing, yet under use, of numerical data. Computers are extremely useful for the retrospective analysis of practice activity, but the data still has to be evaluated and the remainder of the audit cycle carried out, including planning change and setting target standards.

Evaluating information

Once information about an aspect of care has been collected the next step is to consider what it means. It is important to check that the data on which the practice is about to base care decisions is believable. This does not mean that it has to be collected with the rigour required of research, but it must be of adequate quality to justify change. The data therefore need to be complete (or be based on an adequate sample); the collection method should be reliable; and any sampling must be unbiased. These topics are discussed fully in Part II, Chapter 6.

If targets have previously been set in the practice then performance can be compared with them—and either changes can be made to improve care, or the targets may need to be altered to be more challenging or more achievable. If targets have not previously been set, this is the time to use a combination of current performance, local comparisons, expert opinion, and the literature to set them.

Planning care and implementing change

The effectiveness of audit in improving patient care has been shown to depend heavily on the effort to produce change—and yet many audits currently carried out in practice omit the crucial stages of implementing change and setting targets.

Delivery of care depends on four main factors: knowledge, skill, attitudes, and organization. Ashbaugh and McKean (1976), in a survey of 5400 patient records, showed that 95 per cent of deficiencies were due to failure of performance rather than of knowledge. Following any evaluation which reveals failure to achieve target standards, the first reaction of a practice should be to ask whether changing the organization of care would remedy the situation: it is likely that it will.

Repeating the cycle

An advantage of the cyclical nature of audit is that before each phase of data collection there is opportunity to review the criteria and target levels of performance.

No part of the audit cycle is more important than any other and the cycle may be entered at any point. For this reason, no item is put at the top of the audit cycle diagram. In practical terms most practices will begin by planning care ('patients do not seem to be getting appointments easily enough, let's redesign the appointment system'). The next most likely entry point is observing practice and collecting data ('patients do not seem to be getting appointments easily enough, let's measure how long they have to wait'). It is relatively uncommon for a practice to begin by setting a standard ('patients don't seem to be getting appointments easily enough, we believe no patient should wait over two days, let's find out how many do').

Conversely, the advantage of the cycle is that, wherever you may enter the cycle, you will be challenged to undertake each item eventually.

WHO IS INVOLVED IN AUDIT?

The Family Health Service Authorities (FHSAs) have a legal obligation to maintain primary health care quality, but it is generally accepted that quality assurance conducted by external review has not been very successful in the past, largely due to lack of commitment on the part of the professionals. There are, however, certain areas where minimum standards can helpfully be monitored by authority, and no doubt the number of such areas where this takes place will steadily increase. The tensions between, and yet scope for, both confidential and external audit will be reviewed in Part I, Chapter 3.

Within primary care, medical audit was first established by doctors reviewing themselves or each other. *Self audit* is, of course, the most confidential form of audit, but perhaps the least likely to provide change. *Peer audit* involves groups either within practices or between practices co-operating to conduct audit of their care. This provides the benefit of other professionals' constructive criticism, and also an economy of scale in developing criteria: but when carried out between practices there may be difficulty in providing uniform data.

Medical Audit Advisory Groups (MAAGs) have a major role to play in medical audit. Although set up by FHSAs they have a statutory obligation to maintain confidentiality of doctors' audit data from the FHSA. As a result of this they are in a strong position to help practices develop confidential medical audit, and improve their care by means of education. A fuller discussion of the potential of MAAGs will be found in Part IV.

CONCLUSION

Quality improvement must be the goal of medical education and service delivery: medical audit is the activity which underpins such improvement. Understanding the nature of audit is the essential first step in assessing its potentials and dangers, learning how to set about it, and undertaking audit in practice. The remainder of this book examines these issues in turn.

GLOSSARY

1. *Quality assurance:* The assessment of the quality of medical care, the efforts to improve the provision of that care, and the procedure to ensure that good quality is maintained.

2. *Medical audit:* The attempt to improve the quality of medical care by measuring the performance of those providing that care, by considering the performance in relation to desired standards, and by improving on this performance.

3. *Element of care:* Any aspect of care into which a topic of care can be broken down.

4. *Indicators of care:* Elements which are important in assessing a topic of care, and which between them cover all important aspects of the care (effectiveness, equity, humanity, and efficiency).

5. *Criterion of care:* An indicator of care defined so precisely that one can say whether it is present or absent.

6. *Level of performance:* A measure of the extent to which a criterion should be achieved or is achieved.

7. *Standard:* A standard for any indicator of care is derived from the criterion together with its level of performance. Thus a *target standard* is derived from the criterion together with a desired level of performance, and an *achieved standard* is derived from the criterion together with the observed level of performance.

8. *Evaluation:* This can now be carried out by comparing the achieved standard of care with the target for each criterion of care.

9. *Quality of care:* For any topic of care, quality is assessed from the standards set and achieved for the various indicators used to assess that topic of care.

10. *Protocol:* A protocol should include *both* a plan for managing care *and* a plan for audit of that care.

11. *Guidelines:* Suggestions for criteria, levels of performance, or management plans which are provided by external authorities as a basis on which practices can develop their own protocols.

REFERENCES

Ashbaugh, D. G. and McKean, R. S. (1976). Continuing medical education: the philosophy and use of audit. *Journal of the American Medical Association*, **236**, 1485–8.

Black, N. (1990). Quality assurance of medical care. *Journal of Public Health Medicine*, **12** (2), 97–104.

British Medical Association (1965). *Charter for the family doctor service*. BMA, London.

Difford, F. (1990). Defining essential data for audit in general practice. *British Medical Journal* **300**, 92–4.

Donabedian, A. (1982). Introduction to *Explorations in quality assessment and monitoring. Vol. 2: The criteria and standards of quality*. Health Administration Press, Ann Arbor.

Donabedian, A. (1986). Criteria and standards for quality assessment and monitoring. *Quality Review Bulletin*, **12**, 99–108.

Grol, R., Mesker, P., and Schellevis, F. (eds) (1988). *Peer review in general practice*. Nijmegen University Department of General Practice, Nijmegen.

Marinker, M. (ed.) (1990). Medical audit in general practice. *British Medical Journal*.

North of England Study of standards and performance in general practice (1990). Vol. 1. Health Care Research Unit, Newcastle-on-Tyne.

Platt, R. (1967). Medical science. Master or servant? *British Medical Journal*, **4**, 439–44.

Royal College of General Practitioners (1985). *Quality in general practice*. Policy Statement 2. Royal College of General Practitioners, London.

Shaw C. D. (1980). Aspects of audit: the background. *British Medical Journal*, **i**, 1256–8.

Sheldon, M. G. (1982). *Medical audit in general practice*. Occasional Paper 20. Royal College of General Practitioners, London.

2 The purpose of medical audit

Theo Schofield

In 1983 the Royal College of General Practitioners launched its Quality Initiative with the following aims:

1. Each general practitioner should describe his or her current work and should be able to say what services his or her practice provides for the patients.
2. Each general practitioner should define specific objectives for the care of his or her patients and should monitor the extent to which these objectives are met.

One of the central proposals in the British Government's 1989 White Paper on the reform of the National Health Service (NHS) was that all doctors should participate in regular and systematic medical audit (Secretaries of State 1989). This was welcomed by leaders of the medical profession as it was in line with their previously stated policies.

The College and Government gave several reasons for encouraging audit:

- the development of professional education and self-regulation
- improvement of the quality of patient care
- increasing accountability
- improvement of motivation and teamwork
- aiding the assessment of needs
- as a stimulus to research

These are the issues that this chapter considers.

EDUCATION

'To become capable of honesty is the beginning of education' (John Ruskin, *Time and Tide* 1867).

Observing practice

A straightforward descriptive audit can enable us to expose the gap between what we think we do and what we actually do, and can also give us the confidence that we know what we are doing.

Practice activity analysis (Birmingham Research Unit RCGP 1977) started with the collection of data about a particular topic, for example, prescribing or workload. Differences in practice were then used as the starting point for small group discussions which led to the development of criteria for future practice. This method has been shown to be capable of producing change in preventive care where the criteria are relatively non-contentious (Fleming and Lawrence 1983).

Agreeing criteria

Audits which are based on criteria for care involve the process of defining those criteria. We may turn to the relevant medical literature or to experts in this field, or we may discuss our criteria with our colleagues and members of other disciplines and learn from them. It is important that in these discussions firmly held opinions and established wisdom can be challenged. We may also need to be much more explicit about the values that determine some of the choices that we make. Freeling and Burton (1982) described their experiences of performance review in peer groups and identified the need for skilful leadership to avoid the possibility of members joining in a kind of false consensus in order to avoid confrontation with colleagues in the group.

Setting the educational agenda

Each stage in the audit cycle can therefore be of educational value. Another major benefit of audit is its potential for setting the agenda for our continued education and learning. As learners, much of our choice of reading and courses is directed to those areas in which we are already knowledgeable and interested, rather than to those areas of educational need. The same dilemma is also faced by those who provide courses and other education. The value of both audit and continued medical education would be greatly increased if the links between the two were strengthened. This might operate at the individual or practice level by creating a learning plan, either to correct deficiencies in care, or to implement changes agreed as a result of an audit.

At a district level, courses can be provided as a response to problems identified by audit, for example, by providing a course on joint injection techniques to reduce rheumatology referrals.

MOTIVATION AND TEAMWORK

Most aspects of care in general practice involve important contributions, not just from doctors, but also from practice nurses, reception and clerical staff, and other members of a wider team. If a topic is chosen for audit, and all team members are involved in the process of choosing criteria and planning the audit, this will convey the message that their contribution and opinions are valued. It will also increase commitment both to conducting the audit and to responding to its results. During these discussions the aims of care and the values that underpin them can also be shared, which will help to develop a sense of common purpose within the team.

When the results of the audit are shared with the team the rules for feedback which have been developed in other contexts are equally important (Pendleton *et al.* 1984). The strengths that the audit reveals should be discussed first; individuals should be asked to comment on their own performance and acknowledge their own weaknesses, and problems should be discussed not as criticisms but as indications for constructive change. Adhering to these rules has a number of benefits. Identifying strengths and progress, particularly when the targets have already been set, helps to maintain motivation. Open acknowledgement of deficiencies, particularly by the doctors in the team, encourages open communication and the acknowledgement of difficulties by other team members. If the audit generates real changes then the whole exercise will feel worthwhile. Adhering to these rules reinforces and helps people to build on their strengths, and makes critical comment not only more acceptable but also more effective.

IMPROVING QUALITY OF PATIENT CARE

It is by no means automatic that conducting audits will lead to improvement in patient care, and many published studies do not include a repeat audit to demonstrate change (Baker 1990). Grol *et al.* (1988) described the effects of an intensive structured programme of peer review on the behaviour of general practitioners. After taking part in the programme their work conformed more closely to a number of criteria for good general practice care, including aspects of their consultations and prescribing, and the greatest change occurred amongst general practitioners who previously conformed least with the established criteria. Anderson *et al.* (1988) reported a group of general practitioners who studied their prescribing of digoxin and created a protocol which was distributed to their practices. They re-audited their performance one year later. There had been a significant improvement in the group of principals carrying out the audit, but not in the other principals in those practices.

Similar reservations about the effectiveness of audit have been expressed in a number of other reviews (Mitchell and Fowkes 1985; Baker 1991). The conclusions from these is that feedback of information on clinical practice was most likely to influence clinical practice if it was directed to doctors who had already agreed to review their practice, and who were actively involved in setting standards and discussing their performance. Feedback was also more effective if it was immediate and repeated.

The process of planning care and creating protocols which are soundly based will improve care only as long as the plans are adhered to in practice. The likelihood of this happening will be greatly increased if those involved in the delivery of care are also involved in the planning and in agreeing the criteria for the audit. This involvement, by enhancing education, motivation, and teamwork, can also improve care in less tangible ways. The resultant friendliness, enthusiasm, communication, and caring in the team may not be easily measured, but can undoubtedly be perceived by the patients.

The traditional style of quality assurance is of management by exception, in which one only responds to failures or deviations from agreed criteria. In some instances this may be appropriate; for example, a practice whose policy is that no patient requesting an appointment that day should be refused it without the staff consulting a doctor would wish to establish the circumstances if this had occurred. A second style is to set targets and to monitor the extent to which these are achieved. If the practice agrees that no patient should have to wait more than two days for a routine appointment, it is possible to measure how many weeks a year the practice falls short of this and to improve by making changes in the appointment system. Progress is encouraging.

In a more recent approach, described as continuous improvement (Berwick 1989) or 'total quality management', the whole team are committed to continuous monitoring and improvement of their own contribution to the quality of the service, by making changes as and when required. The essential ingredients of this sort of approach, involving the whole team, integrating audit into everyday practice and management, and continuous monitoring and improvement of performance all lead to improvements in quality of patient care.

MANAGEMENT AND ACCOUNTABILITY

In most countries, general practitioners have independence to manage their own practices. They may have to meet certain criteria and achieve particular targets, and the resources that they have available may be limited, but the way in which they plan to meet those criteria and to use those resources remains within their control. As the criteria become more rigorous and the resources more restricted, this management function has become more demanding. It involves defining services to be provided, the quality of the services, and the extent to which that quality is maintained (Irvine 1990). Systematic and regular audit is an essential part of this process, and unless general practitioners become involved, their professional independence will be threatened.

The magnitude of recent change in the services that general practitioners in the UK are expected to provide can hardly be overestimated. From a requirement to deal competently with those patients who present with problems, general practitioners are now expected to provide a comprehensive range of services for the whole practice population. The resources to provide these services are inevitably limited, but a practice's case for any additional support will be greatly strengthened by producing evidence from audits and plans for improvements. Conversely, failure to account for the way the resources have been used may lead to their withdrawal.

NEEDS ASSESSMENT

Thus far audit has been described as looking backwards at aspects of care and making plans to improve that care. Another dimension is to look at the needs of the practice population or groups of patients within it, to identify the extent to which existing services meet those needs, and to make plans to develop those services. In order to be able to assess needs we must define the desired state of health, and determine the degree of shortfall from that state. It is, of course, important to avoid on the one hand setting quite unrealistic goals, such as complete physical, mental, and social well-being for everyone, or on the other hand, choosing minimal goals that fall short of the aspirations of the patients. For example, if one wished to audit the results of a screening programme for elderly patients, realistic goals could be set for freedom from pain, mobility, and independence in activities of daily living. It then becomes possible to assess how many elderly patients do not achieve this goal, and therefore have some health need. It is also important to avoid the trap of equating health need with a need for a particular service. For example, impaired mobility does not equate with the need for total hip replacement, and we must consider a wider range of provision from other members of the primary health care team and other agencies in the community.

The methodology of needs assessment is not well defined, but as it will be the basis for planning and allocating resources in health services in the future, many practice-based audits could start to include this element.

A STIMULUS TO RESEARCH

It is important to distinguish between audit and research. Audit should use established knowledge to assess existing practice, while research aims to collect new knowledge to guide future practice. It might well be, however, that in the process of conducting an audit questions arise to which there are no answers, and some of these then become the subject of research.

There are particular problems in trying to evaluate the effect of changes that have been introduced, because before and after comparisons are commonly made without any control group, and often the numbers in any one practice are too small to demonstrate significant change.

To take one example, if one wished to evaluate the effect of introducing cholesterol screening and dietary advice in a practice it would be quite valid to audit the number of patients who had been screened before and after the introduction of the service as a measure of the process of care. If, on the other hand, one wished to assess the effectiveness of the dietary advice for the patients with elevated cholesterol levels, a control group would be required to allow for the effect of background changes in the population, and for the fact that subsequent readings in patients with elevated levels of cholesterol may be lower by the chance process of regression to the mean. It would also be extremely difficult, if not impossible, to demonstrate the effect of lowering cholesterol on arterial disease in a single practice. In other words, research and audit are enterprises of a totally different magnitude.

RESISTANCE TO AUDIT

If audit is such a desirable activity for practices, why is it not more widely practised? Audit can undoubtedly be seen as complex, and the demands on time may be incompatible with the need to provide patient care. In addition, if the principal purpose of audit is seen to be critical rather than constructive, and if it is thought to be the preserve of a particular elite, it will not gain credibility from local opinion leaders.

The experience of practices which have become involved in auditing their own work suggests that the time involved has paid handsome dividends, both in improved patient care and in increased job satisfaction and team support. There is undoubtedly a political dimension as well. Avedis Donabedian (1986) in his visit to Britain in 1984 found:

In the larger community of practitioners the auditing of performance was valued if it was seen as an anticipatory pre-emptive enterprise capable of mobilising consumers' support and avoiding the need for Government intervention. By contrast auditing was shunned if it seemed to threaten to awaken the sleeping dogs of public discontent or to offer a ready made tool that could be used indiscriminately and oppressively by Government. Often the auditing of performance seems to have been regarded as both hastening and defending against the dangers that the practitioners envisaged, and ambivalence was the consequence of not knowing which of the two effects would dominate.

These fears and this ambivalence persist, but at the present time medical audit remains a professional responsibility and the medical profession has the opportunity of assuring its patients of the quality of the services that it provides. Failure to grasp this opportunity will surely lead to the controls and the loss of independence that the profession fears most. As Donabedian stated, 'this being the case we have no choice but to proceed'.

REFERENCES

Anderson, C. M., Chambers, S., Clamp, M., Dunn, I., McGhee, M., Summer, K., and Wood, A. (1988). Can audit improve patient care: effects of studying use of digoxin in general practice. *British Medical Journal*, **297**, 113–14.

Baker, R. (1990). Problem solving with audit in general practice. *British Medical Journal*, **300**, 378–80.

Baker, R. (1991). Audit and standards in new general practice. *British Medical Journal*, **303**, 32–4.

Berwick, D. M. (1989). Continuous improvement as an ideal in health care. *New England Journal of Medicine*, **320**, 53–6.

The Birmingham Research Unit of the Royal College of General Practitioners. (1977). Self evaluation in general practice. *Journal of the Royal College of General Practitioners*, **27**, 265–70.

Donabedian, A. (1986). Impressions of a journey in Britain. *In pursuit of quality* (ed. D. Pendleton, T. Schofield, and M. Marinker), pp. 146–67. Royal College of General Practitioners, London.

Fleming, D. M. and Lawrence, M. S. (1983). Impact of audit on preventive measures. *British Medical Journal*, **287**, 1852–4.

Freeling, P. and Burton, R. H. (1982). General practitioners and learning by audit. *Journal of the Royal College of General Practitioners*, **32**, 231–7.

Grol, R., Mokkink, H., and Schellevis, F. (1988). The effects of peer review in general practice. *Journal of the Royal College of General Practitioners*, **38**, 10–13.

Irvine, D. (1990). *Managing for quality in general practice*. King's Fund Centre, London.

Mitchell, M. W. and Fowkes, F. G. R. (1985). Audit reviewed: does feedback on performance change clinical behaviour? *Journal of the Royal College of Physicians London*, **19**, 251–4.

Pendleton, D., Schofield, T., Tate, P., and Havelock, P. (1984). *The consultation: an approach to learning and teaching*. Oxford University Press.

Royal College of General Practitioners. (1983). The quality initiative. *Journal of the Royal College of Practitioners*, **33**, 523–4.

Secretaries of State for Health, Wales, Northern Ireland and Scotland (1989). *Working for patients*. HMSO, London.

3 Medical audit and accountability

David Metcalfe

To be an independent contractor is not to be absolved of accountability. Doctors are paid to provide medical care, and many of the actions they take cost the NHS public money. Those who spend public money are accountable to Ministers in Parliament. In the case of primary health care this accountability is mediated through Family Health Service Authorities (FHSAs), who supervise contracts by monitoring claims for item of service or target achievement, prescribing activity from Prescribing Analysis and Cost (PACT), and now other activities from practice reports. This constitutes external performance review, and it enables FHSAs to make comparisons, both between practices and between any given practice and whatever it chooses to cite as the 'norm' or expected level of performance.

ACCOUNTABILITY BY EXTERNAL MONITORING

Some points about external performance review or monitoring should be borne in mind. First, only relatively discrete and clearly defined actions, such as immunizations, prescriptions, investigations, or referrals, are amenable to it (and, apart from prescribing, such actions account for a relatively small proportion of all the clinical activity that general practitioners are involved in). Because they are discrete, their performance is measured, or more properly counted, on a 'two-point' scale: either it was done or it was not done.

Secondly, external monitoring is not amenable to shades of meaning; nor can it make allowances for professional judgement or the effect of intervening factors. It is a relatively blunt instrument for assessing performance in such a complex activity as general practice.

Thirdly, it is essentially a management tool, and tools are, by definition, for use. Management tools are used by managers, and the way that they use them reflects a manager's way of looking at things. Almost all surveys of general pactice activity have shown wide variations in the pattern of care provided. They can be presented as distribution curves, and are characteristically wide and flat. Managers prefer activity distribution curves which are tall and narrow: these describe fairly standard, and therefore predictable, behaviour. They cannot believe that two doctors whose referral rates vary by a factor of four can possibly be providing equally effective and economical care. They would like there to be 'norms' of performance to which individual practices' activities could be compared, and anyone deviating too far from the norm subjected to corrective procedures, whether of the stick or carrot variety. Unfortunately, there are few norms (such as achievement of immunization coverage) that can be justified in terms of cost-effective care: no-one, for example, can define the 'right' referral rate. When it comes to making comparisons between practices, the bluntness of external performance review, using routinely collected data, makes it impossible to be sure that like is being compared with like.

In terms of FHSA activity, the word 'audit' should be reserved for its precise commercial use: a searching examination by outsiders to deter or detect fraud, to make sure that what is being claimed for has actually been done.

External performance review, using routinely collected data from all the practices within an FHSA area, has to be seen as a normal management procedure to which contracting practices must be prepared to submit. It is nothing new: the new contract merely extends its scope. It should not be called audit because it is not an individual enquiry or examination undertaken for a specific purpose, and the idea of being 'audited' by the FHSA generates anxiety and resentment in contracting practitioners. It has several limitations, and it is important that managers do not over-interpret its results.

The fallacy of the industrial analogy

Terms such as audit, performance review, and quality assurance have been brought into health services from industry and commerce together with the doctrines of the market. Before adopting them it is worth considering the fact that the conceptual model of industry is not really applicable to a health service. Industry buys raw material, processes it with energy and expertise, and sells the finished product. Some of the selling price goes back to purchase more raw material and energy and invest in more expertise, the rest is distributed to the shareholders as profit. Illness cannot really be seen as a raw material, and the end product, which is usually decreased or controlled ill health rather than complete health, is not saleable.

Nor does the model of a 'service' industry correspond to health services. Service industry responds to demand not need (who *needs* a ride on a roller coaster?), and deliberately creates demand by advertizing. Their customers *choose* to buy their services.

Other concepts from commerce also fail to transplant. In business it is supposed to be fatal to be reactive: to survive a business must be proactive, seeing new market opportunities and going for them. Health services are now enjoined to be proactive not reactive, but if the negatively charged word 'reactive' is replaced by the more positively charged word 'responsive' the message feels quite different: surely health services must respond to needs presented to them? Proactive in health services has been allowed, unchallenged, to become equated with preventive: health service managers and their political overlords want to *avoid* business. In their terms proactive certainly does not mean planning for more transplant surgery for an ageing population.

'Quality' in industry and commerce focuses on acceptability: does the product satisfy the customers' wants enough to ensure that they come back to buy more goods or services? Quality in medical care addresses four concerns: is the care effective, economical, acceptable, and equitable (i.e., is it equally available to all, regardless of age, gender, socioeconomic status, or ethnicity?) The aim in providing quality is to reduce the need for more care. For these reasons concepts from industry and commerce, from which health professionals can benefit, need to be subjected to critical assessment before being adopted as a basis for policy.

ACCOUNTABILITY BY MEDICAL AUDIT

If external monitoring is the way in which FHSAs are entitled and able to exercise accountability, it can be seen to be concerned with the question 'How *much*?'. Professionals have accountability in two other dimensions however: to their clients, and to their colleagues, and their question is 'How *well*?'. Doctors, like members of the other learned professions, give *advice* to their clients, rather than orders.

Doctors should explain the problem to patients, allow them to make informed choices, and then support them in the choice they make. The advice must be given in good faith, and the trust that this is so is an essential ingredient of the doctor-patient relationship. That trust generates the question 'How well did he or she do it?'.

Poor performance, things not being done as well as they should and could be, reflects not only on the trustworthiness of the individual doctor concerned but, by extrapolation, on the rest of the profession. It is important to understand that there are preconceived adverse feelings about all professionals in society at large: they have power, they share the mystery of their craft, and they are well rewarded for their labours. Individual episodes of poor performance therefore are used to justify and reinforce these negative feelings. To provide poor care therefore not only puts the patient at risk and forfeits his or her trust, but damages the standing of the profession at large. Hence, accountability to colleagues also implies asking the question 'How well?'.

A true profession is self-policing, since by definition it is concerned with matters that cannot be fully understood by lay people. From Hippocrates onward there has been a requirement for altruism: the willingness to 'put oneself out' to a lesser or greater degree for the benefit of a patient or patients. As evidence a wide range of self-sacrifice can be cited, from waiving of fees at one end, through self-experimentation, to innumerable examples of doctors actually losing their lives in attempting to save others. In part this may be specific to medicine because of the sanctity of life, but in part it may reflect the consciousness that, nowadays at least, the profession is held in high esteem and well rewarded by society, and that such privileges have to be earned or paid for.

Professionalism, in both of these senses, demands of doctors a determination to do the job as well as they can, and ensure that their colleagues do too. Clinical audit by peer review should have always been a natural component of medical practice: now it is enjoined upon it in NHS regulations.

PROBLEMS WITH MEDICAL AUDIT AS A MEANS OF ACCOUNTABILITY

Peer review by clinical audit, as a professional responsibility, faces a variety of problems which should deter both doctors, managers, and their political masters from a simplistic approach. These problems fall into two main categories: that of scientific philosophy; and that of operational considerations.

Problems with the scientific philosophy of medical audit

There are two main difficulties about asking 'How well?'. The first is the definition of 'good' care and the criteria for whether it is done 'well'. The second is that really good care, being person-centred, will vary from patient to patient.

Good care comprises all the components of quality: effectiveness, acceptability, economy, and equity. Obviously if care is not effective its acceptability, economy, and equity are irrelevant, and confirming effectiveness is complicated by the fact that there is often only a tenuous connection between the process of care and its outcome. Of course, in some conditions and situations the connection is demonstrably close and direct: patients whose signs and symptoms conform to a protocol for acute appendicitis are much more likely to survive if they have an appendicectomy; people with diabetes are much less likely to go blind if their optic fundi are properly inspected at regular intervals. But many of the patterns of care which are held to be 'good medicine' have never been proved to be effective, either because the benefit was held to be self-evident, and so never tested, or because research has been undertaken and the results proved inconclusive. Quite often the pundits' assertions have, in fact, later been reversed by research; for instance low residue diets for inflammatory bowel disease, or long-term anticoagulants for people who have suffered myocardial infarction.

This is particularly true in general practice where the patient's dis-ease is not well defined and there are multiple interventions (was it being taken seriously, or getting a clear explanation, or the drug prescribed, or the offer of follow-up which made the patient feel better?). Much general practice care is concerned with chronic disease, where the desired outcome is not cure but changes in the gradient of deterioration, or avoidance of complications which might not have happened anyway. Prudence would dictate that outcomes should be measured or assessed long enough after an intervention to give it time to work or its side effects to become apparent; but the longer the interval, outside the relatively controlled environment of the hospital, the more likely it is that intervening variables will affect the outcome one way or the other.

Some interventions have costs even when they achieve their primary objective (protecting a hypertensive person from stroke may make him impotent, or even increase his risk of having a myocardial infarction): what is 'good' care for the condition may be 'not so good' for the patient.

This presents the second problem with regard to the scientific philosophy of audit: can it reflect the subtleties of patient-centred care? Put another way, can a 'criterion of care' be developed which is sensitive to variations in patient characteristics? The 'proper' management of urinary tract infection, for example, is not the same in a 15-year-old boy and a 95-year-old woman. General practitioners are often judged, and found wanting, by surgeons and their registrars, when they send in a patient with suspected appendicitis without doing a rectal examination. Such an invasive procedure may have discriminatory power with regard to the urgency of surgery in the admitted patient. If it is not discriminatory in a patient with enough other signs to justify admission, it is not part of 'good' care in general practice.

The scientific and philosophical problems with audit can therefore be summed up in the following way:

1. Where process has been shown to be clearly related to outcome, valid criteria for care can be promulgated: failure to achieve a high level of performance would be to put patients at risk.
2. Where process has not been shown to be clearly related to outcome the criteria can only be described as 'state-of-the-art', and achievement of high level of performance represents only conformity with current professional opinion. Low levels of performance do not necessarily put patients at risk.
3. State-of-the-art criteria therefore have to be amenable to adjustment for patient and situational factors.
4. Criteria validated by outcome can be used to indicate effectiveness; state-of-the-art criteria indicate both conformity with conventional wisdom and sensitivity to patients and their situations, and sometimes these are in conflict with each other.

Problems with the operation of medical audit

The other category of problems faced by those undertaking peer review by medical audit is that of operational considerations: what to audit, how extensively, and how often? Unless the magnitude of the problem is appreciated there is a danger of believing that accountability can only be satisfied if every aspect of care is reviewed in the whole practice regularly.

General practitioners provide preventive, acute, chronic, and terminal care to registered populations which are heterogeneous in terms of demographic and socio-economic characteristics. It seems to have become automatic to think of audit as cohort studies of process in patients with chronic disease. Diabetes and hypertension are firm favourites for early efforts at audit within practices. Cohort studies are, by definition, numerate: the same data set is collected from as many people in the cohort as possible, so that the level of performance can be described as a rate. But even in the chronic diseases consideration should be given to what to audit. It is of little value, for example, to audit the fundoscopy rate in a practice diabetic clinic if few of the diabetic patients have even been diagnosed as such, or if large numbers of elderly patients with the disease cannot attend the sessions.

Again, it seems to have become accepted that audit addresses process, while critical examination of structure ('Are our nurses doing work that a receptionist could do?') or outcome ('Is our coronary death rate higher than expected for a population like ours?') are either not seen as audit at all or too difficult. It is often said that using deaths, or standardized mortality ratios, as a basis for audit would not be worthwhile in general practice, since the number of avoidable or preventable deaths in the average practice population is very small: the mistake is to assume that the audit approach must be quantitative. It could be qualitative, whereby every untoward event triggers a case study: 'With hindsight could we have done better?' (see Chapter 13).

Cohort studies of patients with relatively common conditions involve quite large numbers of patients whose records must be reviewed or who may have to be called in for interview or specific tests, or have questionnaires sent to them (in a practice with 10 000 registered patients it is expected that there will be nearly 200 diabetic patients). What are the opportunity costs of plodding through all those frustratingly incomplete records? Would a survey of a sample suffice, and if so, how big a sample and how should it be drawn? (see Chapter 6).

Lastly, the 'audit cycle' has been well publicized, but at what interval after changes are made in response to the findings of a primary audit should the secondary audit be done? The whole of a practice's audit activity after a few years might be taken up by secondary or tertiary audits even though many other aspects of care have never been subjected to primary audit.

The operational problems of audit demand that it is a planned activity with clear objectives and a programme to achieve them. A powerful basis for such a plan would be a matrix approach, combining structure, process, and outcome on one axis, with preventive, acute, chronic, and terminal care on the other. In each of the boxes so formed audit questions should be formulated. Audit questions must be precise. It is unhelpful to say 'We will look at our hypertensive patients': an estimate of prevalence would be an audit of diagnostic inquisitiveness; an enquiry into the incidence of impotence would be an audit of prescribing responsibility; an analysis of recorded blood pressures would be an audit of effectiveness; and a case study of every stroke patient an audit of many aspects of care—was the diagnosis early enough, was the work up complete, was the treatment appropriate and acceptable, were complications avoided, was quality of life maintained? Precise audit questions keep the scale of audits manageable and economic. They also facilitate prioritization: 'What are the features of this practice that indicate an urgent need to find out what is going on?'

MEDICAL AUDIT AND EXTERNAL ACCOUNTABILITY— A MAAG COMPROMISE?

Governments and NHS managers, well aware of wide variations in process, and some variation in outcome, have long craved after the exercise of power over the clinical activity of their doctors, but have been frustrated by the recognition that only peer review is likely to be valid, let alone politically acceptable. The inception of audit as a service-wide activity, and very considerable investment in it, represent what must be seen as a genuine advance toward professional responsibility. In general practice, although audit is not an activity demanded by the new contract, Medical Audit Advisory Groups (MAAGs) have been set up and comparatively well resourced in order to stimulate and facilitate audit in each FHSA area. The emphasis has been placed on it being peer-led, and in most regions the need for separation from management performance review (and hence distancing it from FHSA premises, staff, and data) has been clearly recognized and respected. MAAG chairpersons have to report to FHSA chairs and their general managers on the extent of audit among their general practice contractors, and this is generally taken to mean the proportion of general practitioners who are undertaking audit, the range of topics audited, and the frequency with which audits have resulted in change. (The subject of MAAGs is discussed more fully in Chapter 20.)

The MAAG programme therefore offers several benefits to FHSAs, their general practice contractors, and the people in their registered populations. At the practice level, getting general practitioners to look critically at their own care will help them to close what may be the biggest gap, that between what they honestly think they are doing and what they actually *are* doing. At the district level, by discussing the levels of performance expected among practices auditing the same topic, MAAGs can contribute to a harmonization of standards. Practices will, in the first place, set their own standards in the light of what seems to them to be appropriate and achievable. Knowing what standards other practices have set for the same topic may well cause them to revise their own. MAAGs will also have the opportunity to institute 'area wide' audits in which a large number of practices carry out audits on the same topic, or on various aspects of it. So far such initiatives mostly seem to have come from within the MAAG, often from its specialist members, and reflect the clinical interests of those members. This may or may not address local problems that should have priority. In time, however, it can also be expected that MAAGs will be prepared to facilitate area-wide audits in response to concerns arising outwith its membership and transmitted to its chairperson by others, such as FHSA officers,

Directors of Public Health, Community Health Councils, hospital specialists, general practitioners themselves, lay groups, or others.

Problems of interpractice comparisons

These opportunities for MAAGs seem to be widely appreciated and to inform much of their early work and planning. But the idea of area-wide audits illustrates a danger which has to be faced. If such an enquiry gets general practitioners to examine their clinical care for a certain topic, compare it with reasonably harmonized target standards, and consider what changes to make to enable them to reach a higher level of achievement, it will have succeeded in what should have been its objectives. If, however, the detailed results of each practice's audit are collected, collated, and analysed in an attempt to describe the process of care across the FHSA area, dangers become apparent. Were the practices representative of the whole area? Did each datum describe the same action or item of care, and were there agreed definitions for this? (An estimate of HbA1c is a 'yes or no' event, but a recording of dorsalis pedis pulse palpability depends on the doctor's skill as well as his or her willingness to make the examination. Depth of depression is even more vulnerable to the personal equation, but may be an important observation in an audit of the effectiveness of care). Multi-observer research has to put a great deal of effort not only into defining every relevant term, but training the observers to adhere to them and checking that they do. There would have to be agreement as to inclusion and exclusion criteria lest bias creep in. Area-wide audit is unlikely to be resourced to do that. Without these precautions the results of practice audits cannot reliably be combined to describe the totality of care in the area, let alone to compare practices or put them in rank order. The desire for area-wide descriptions of process, and rank-ordering of practices is essentially a management instinct to reduce variation, and that could not be justified unless the results were as valid and reliable as those from formal research.

Another technical problem with pooling data from individual audits concerns the denominators used to describe rates or proportions. To say that '90 per cent of our diabetic patients had fundoscopy last year' depends for its value on the meaning of 'our diabetic patients': if they represent the expected 2 per cent of the population that is a highly desirable achievement; if they represent only half the expected number it is much less so. The validity of process rates depends on the completeness of identification of the cohort, and the representativeness of any sample on which the audit was based.

Comparisons of process and outcome can only be made if events are reduced to rates. Examples would be deaths per 100 000 people, or investigations per 100 consultations. But the choice of denominator is not always obvious or simple. For example, Table 3.1 describes four doctors' referral characteristics and shows the effect of using different denominators. It can be seen that changing the denominator changes the rank order of resource utilization—

Table 3.1 *Referral characteristics for four doctors each with 2000 registered patients*

Doctor	Consultation rate (contacts/patient/year)	Consultations per year	Number of people consulting in one year and percentage of practice population	Number of referrals	Rates (and rank order)		
					Referrals per 1000 people on list	Referrals per 100 consultations	Referrals per 1000 people who consult
A	2.8	5600	1340 (67%)	450	225 (4)	8 (1)	336 (2)
B	3.1	6200	1400 (70%)	460	230 (3)	7.5 (2)	329 (3)
C	3.4	6800	1350 (67.5%)	470	235 (2)	7 (3)	348 (1)
D	3.7	7400	1500 (75%)	480	240 (1)	6.5 (4)	320 (4)

indeed in this example changing from referrals per 1000 patients on the list to referrals per 100 consultations reversed the order. Which doctor does have the most appropriate referral behaviour?

The problems that arise when audit data are collected from the practices, pooled, collated, and analysed, even within the confidentiality of the MAAG, are those inherent in epidemiological and health services research. Is like being compared with like? Has everybody adhered to the procedures laid down? Are the denominators the correct ones for the audit question being addressed?

Audit is not research: those auditing themselves and each other are neither trained nor resourced to undertake research, and the opportunity costs in terms of other audits would be too high if they tried. It is sometimes objected that if audit cannot be done to research standards it should not be done at all because the results are not reliable enough to be useful. This is true if the findings are held to be generalizable and used for policy making outside the practices. But *inside* the practices there is less danger of like not being compared with like, or of wide differences in definitions and adherence to agreed procedures. Findings which could not justifiably be generalized outside to other practices and other places *can* be used as stimuli for change inside the practice. While many of the methods are common to both audit and research, the level of precision needed is not. Thus a research project which failed to collect data from 30 per cent of the possible subjects would be seen as a failure because of the likelihood of bias arising from the non-responders. An audit project, on the other hand, which encountered the same problem would achieve two objectives: 70 per cent of the possible subjects would get their care reviewed and where necessary improved; and the difficulty in identifying the other 30 per cent, or getting data from their records, would have been identified as a problem which must be solved.

CONCLUSION

In summary it could be said that acceptance of contract monitoring comes with appointment to a clinical post, but acceptance of medical audit should come with the medical degree. Each addresses different aspects of professional accountability, at different levels of meaning and precision. Contract supervision is too blunt and crude an instrument for accountability to patients and colleagues. Professional review will be effective as an agent of change within practices even if it forgoes research precision, even though this makes it too imprecise as an instrument of accountability to managers.

We are left with a two track model for audit and accountability. Doctors can expect and accept external performance review as their accountability to managers, and beyond them, to Ministers in Parliament. But they are also accountable to their patients and their colleagues, and must not only accept but actively promote peer review to give that accountability meaning. The way to do that is by planned programmes of audit.

Part II
Establishing audit in primary health care

Introduction: Preparing the ground

Peter Havelock

The introduction of audit into a practice can be fraught with difficulties. To maximize the chances of success an essential first step is for the practice team to take an inward look to see if it is capable of and ready for the challenge. The mood of the whole practice needs to be right. Successful audit requires members of the team to have confidence in each other, an ability to work together, enthusiasm and energy, the ability to accept criticism, and a wish to improve.

It is not always possible to produce entirely the right mood in the practice before starting audit. Sometimes there are seemingly insuperable obstacles. For instance, a difficult partner or practice manager, an overwhelming workload, or terrible premises, can make individuals feel discouraged before starting. But it is quite feasible to start in a very modest way, either alone or with another person of like mind. Looking at the quality of care and trying to improve it can be an introduction to a whole new way of working in the practice. Audit can often be the first truly shared activity in the practice and many others can follow.

As a practice goes ahead with medical audit three fundamental questions need to be answered:

1. What kind of practice are we?
2. What kind of practice do we want to be?
3. How capable of change are we?

This approach is not new. Work has already been undertaken in industry which can help formulate answers to these questions (Stewart 1972). In this chapter some of those established principles are applied to general practice. Just as it helps to look at our patients and define them in terms of health or ill-health, so too we can look at our practices and ask the same questions: What makes a healthy practice team? What makes a healthy organization?

A HEALTHY PRACTICE IS PURPOSEFUL, IT 'KNOWS WHERE IT IS GOING'

In general practice all members rarely agree on the direction in which the practice is going. We probably all agree that attending to the patients who walk in through the door is our main purpose, but a healthy practice also has a shared view on prevention, chronic disease management, involvement of the practice in the community, teaching strategy, and so on. In particular, a healthy practice needs a shared view on its purpose in undertaking audit, and how quality improvement fits into each area of medical care.

A HEALTHY PRACTICE IS GROUNDED IN REALITY

This is not usually a problem with general practice because of the urgent and immediate demands of dealing with patients. Even so, a practice can easily become unaware of, or unresponsive to, the needs of the patients. For example, this may result in:

(1) not enough appointments;
(2) not enough telephone lines;
(3) not enough space.

A HEALTHY PRACTICE HAS OPEN COMMUNICATION

Open communication means that everyone within the organization has a mechanism for communicating easily with all others within that organization, and is able to use it. It also means that there is a minimum of secretive communication, and then only when it is necessary to protect individuals.

Within practices the communication between partner and partner, doctor and employed staff, and attached staff and the core team is often minimal and closed. A healthy practice has defined and easy access to the doctors by all staff, with regular meetings for education and sharing information.

IN A HEALTHY PRACTICE REWARD IS LINKED TO ACHIEVEMENT

Reward is not solely financial, but includes other rewards for the recognition of good work. The financial reward should be sufficient recompense for the work done within the recognized guidelines of a job, but other rewards can often be a more significant motivating factor.

Maslow (1954), in his hierarchy of needs (Fig. 1), suggests that once the basic needs for food, shelter, and security are met, other needs play a greater part in motivating people. It is difficult for people to feel good about themselves if they are poorly paid, are under threat, and have no respect within work. But the social needs of being valued and being part of a team, and the ego needs of growth and development become important rewards once the lower order needs have been fulfilled.

In terms of a healthy practice, achievement can be recognized in a number of ways—a sufficient and equitable pay structure, pleasant and suitable working

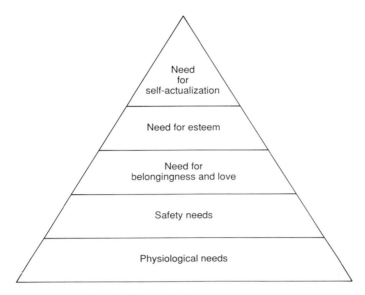

Fig. 1 Maslow's hierarchy of needs.

conditions, an atmosphere of mutual support, appropriate delegation of responsibility, and social activity, such as a Christmas party or summer barbeque.

IN A HEALTHY PRACTICE DECISIONS ARE MADE AT THE LOWEST POSSIBLE LEVEL

The lowest possible level means that level which is closest to the area of work
that the decision affects. In large organizations this can mean the delegation of
decision-making on day-to-day running to the managers who are responsible for
the implementation of those decisions.

In terms of general practice, it means letting those members of staff who are
responsible for certain parts of the practice take decisions about them. For
instance, the practice nurse may review the different makes of sterilizer and
other equipment and propose purchase; or the secretaries may make their own
decisions about typewriters, facsimile machines, and office procedures, and
make proposals to the partners.

IN A HEALTHY PRACTICE LEADERSHIP IS VISIBLE

In industry this is 'management by wandering around', with encouragement of
managers to have their office doors open, offering easy access for discussion and
consultation.

In practice, similar principles apply. The doctors make the management decisions and they must be accessible to all members, so the gap between 'leaders' and 'workers' is as small as possible.

A HEALTHY PRACTICE MANAGES ITS BOUNDARIES

A healthy organization is aware of what is within and what is outside its organization, and makes the distinction clear, so that everyone knows where they stand. Within general practice, because the organization is small, this should be easy, but those on the boundary (for example, the community psychiatric nurse, the school nurse or the social worker) may not know clearly either the appropriate channels of communication or their relationships with the practice.

SUMMARY

It can be very helpful to view general practice in the same way in which management consultants view organizations. We can use the lessons that have been well tried in industry to improve our practices. We can change from an 'unhealthy practice' to a 'healthy practice'. A healthy practice will find any change, including audit, easier and less traumatic to doctors and staff. It is worthwhile looking at those factors which tend to result in healthy organizations and see if our practices can adopt them.

REFERENCES

Maslow, A. (1954). *Motivation and personality*. Harper, London.
Stewart, R. (1972). *The reality of organisations*. McMillan Pan, London.

4 Choosing the topic and getting started

Martin Lawrence

> The Centipede was happy quite
> Until the Toad in fun said
> 'Pray which leg goes after which?'
> Which worked her mind to such a pitch
> She lay distracted in the ditch
> Considering how to run.

Starting an audit can feel like a major decision. Will it be a lot of work? Will it be worth the effort? Should we not rather be looking at something else? Are we ready to take it on? Should we not first get more staff, or better records? There are always plenty of uncertainties, plenty of reasons for putting things off. This not only applies to the *first* audit. Practices who have already embarked on audit still face the same decisions when it comes to taking on a new topic—What shall we drop?, Is this particular topic the next most important?, and so on. We need to get past the 'blocks' and have some guidelines as to where our efforts may be most worthwhile.

BLOCKS TO GETTING STARTED

Time

Every general practitioner is busy, and so are their staff. Audit activity can be seen as yet another call on time in a busy day, and one which diminishes, rather than increases, patient contact. It is a fear exacerbated by reading large audits performed and reported in journals, and reinforced because the data collection exercises demanded by the 1990 general practice contract have been so extensive. But no company would sacrifice the quality control of its products because it wants to spend more time making them: and nor can we sacrifice quality assurance to increased activity.

There are several ways of overcoming the time problem.

1. *Keep it small and simple (KISS)*. This can be achieved by using a small sample to examine a large topic—such as drawing 10 sets of records to assess a health promotion clinic; or by tackling a small topic, for example the control of patients on anticoagulants. The practice may then decide to do a larger study to answer any questions that this first study may raise.

2. *Start by example*. If the enthusiast in a practice — general practitioner, nurse, or practice manager — can do a simple audit and demonstrate that it was not too time consuming, then others may join in. There is a danger that enthusiasts may be left doing the audits on their own, partly because that is convenient for the rest of the practice, and partly because they may have difficulty in letting go. It is important that this should not happen: it deprives the rest of the team of the stimulus of participating, and even enthusiasts run out of energy and become a rate-limiting step in the process.
3. *Work together*. If an audit is planned by a team, then the work can be spread to use everyone's skills and share the time taken. Traditionally this has been done by delegation, with doctors or practice manager planning the audit and staff collecting the data. But if the whole team is involved at the planning stage there will be a much greater feeling of ownership and motivation, and the data collection will probably be carried out more fully and willingly.

Records and computers

'We cannot do an audit because our practice is buying a computer and it's only just arrived'. It is good to have good records, this makes it easier to find necessary information; and of course it is good to have a computer — relevant patients can be identified more easily, and in some cases the required information can be obtained directly from the machine. But computer information is in no way necessary for audit, and may indeed be obstructive.

It is a common misapprehension that audit can be carried out by conducting a computer search and printing out data. The topics that are suitable for data collection by computer may not be those which the practice team feels are most important for audit. There is a danger that items of little interest are reviewed simply because the data are available. A great deal of information needed for audit is not adequately recorded by computers, so a note search may still be required: and it is increasingly appreciated that many valuable audits involve small samples or do not involve numerical analysis at all.

Even if the topic is suitable for computer analysis, that still only completes the data collection element of the cycle. The results still need to be discussed and evaluated so that change can be implemented. Perhaps the most common deficiency in audit work is to restrict the activity to collecting the data and discussing it among the doctors, setting no targets and making no changes.

The practice team

It helps to have a high level of staffing, for the practice manager to be trained in audit, or to employ a records officer. But if we wait for this ideal situation to be present in the practice, many of us will wait for a very long time. Simple audits can be carried out by individuals or groups, and then presented to the rest of the practice team members. Indeed, such activity may be a powerful stimulus to team building, which will make the exercise easier as time goes on.

HELP IN GETTING STARTED

The Medical Audit Advisory Group (MAAG)

These groups, established by every FHSA under the 1990 contract, exist to stimulate and develop audit in the FHSA area. They employ visiting teams, co-ordinators or facilitators, and usually also have a resource office with an administrator. They operate on a confidential basis and are dedicated to helping practices at all levels of audit activity from the simple to the more advanced. Any practice wishing to embark on an audit and unsure of the best methods would be well advised to contact its local MAAG for help (see Chapter 20).

Other people and bodies willing to help will include local practices which may have suitable protocols and be willing to share (the MAAG may well put practices in touch): the general practitioner tutor at the local postgraduate centre: or the audit fellow of the Royal College of General Practitioners (RCGP).

Written or computer-based audit protocols

These are increasingly available. Again, the RCGP Audit Office can help: the RCGP Research Unit, Birmingham, produces practice activity analysis sheets which can be used by practices wishing to collect data on a variety of topics (Crombie and Fleming 1988) (Fig. 4.1): several books include guidelines (for example, the practice audit plan) (Baker and Presley 1990): and increasingly general practice computer systems are providing screen templates which enable practices to collect and analyse data on topics such as preventive care and chronic disease management (Lawrence *et al.* 1990).

GETTING STARTED — A PRACTICE MEETING

The need to work as a team has been emphasized, and the prerequisites of a healthy team outlined in the previous chapter. That team now needs to be prepared to undertake audit.

Many of the team will have no concept of the nature of audit, what it means, what it involves, or why it is necessary. They may feel put upon by work or threatened by performance review. It is necessary to meet and discuss openly many of the principles and purposes of audit. This may be just as important for practices which already do audit as for those just beginning — many practices do audit with most of the staff entirely ignorant of what is going on and why. It is never too late to begin the process of communication. Somebody will need to take the lead, usually either a partner or a practice manager, because there will be need both for teaching and the enabling of open and free discussion. Certain topics have to be covered:

What audit is

This is very much a matter of sharing with the whole team the substance of Part I of this book. In particular the whole team must appreciate that the aim is to identify areas for improvement, and make changes for the better, on a confidential basis. They need to see that the results should be better care for patients, but also improved morale and motivation for themselves. It is necessary for them to understand that there is some work involved, but that everyone will be sharing and that appropriate time will be made available. No benefit will occur unless information is shared, plans are made and change takes place, so it is important that meetings are held for feedback and that everyone who can attends.

What audit is not

It is equally important to discuss the threats implied by audit. It may be the first time that many of the team have had their work examined, and the immediate feeling is that it will be to find fault. The principle of confidentiality will need to be established, and reassurance given that more is likely to be revealed that is good than bad. The principle must be established that in any review the good points will be drawn out first, emphasizing strengths, and only then will the weaknesses be reviewed—and any deficiency will only be discussed in the context of a constructive plan for change.

The principle of participation

Audit is quality assurance carried out by those personally involved in the delivery of care. Just as general practitioners feel threatened by external monitoring and can make better changes by internal audit, so staff will not wish to be audited by their employers, but will do a better job using peer review. Moreover, the practice needs participation, not just to collect the data but to identify topics for audit, areas of difficulty, and methods of improvement. The principles of total quality management are ideally applied to primary care teams, with everyone examining their own particular area of work with an aim to improving its quality.

Agreement will also be needed on how to set up audit teams. Clearly, everyone cannot be involved with every audit, and it will be necessary to agree to set up sub-teams—for example, with three or four people of different disciplines—for any audit topic, with an understanding that the results of any audit are presented to and discussed by the whole primary health care team so that changes and targets can be agreed by everyone.

The Royal College of General Practitioners

PRACTICE ACTIVITY ANALYSIS

11. WORKLOAD REVIEW

This analysis is concerned with aspects of the General Practitioners working week and is measured during a continuous period of two weeks.

A separate sheet is used by each participating doctor and when completed summarise the results in the appropriate places, complete the data return sheet and return the entire document to your group leader or directly to

P.A.A.
RCGP Research Unit
54 Lordswood Road
Birmingham B17 9DB

Page 2 contains the Instructions and Services Provided Score Grid
Page 3 contains the Consultations Table and the Miscellaneous Activity Time Schedule
Page 4 contains the Data Return Sheet

Fig. 4.1 An example of a practice activity analysis.

Page 2

INSTRUCTIONS   SERVICES PROVIDED INDEPENDENT OF CONSULTATION

A score is made every time one of the services listed below is provided for a N.H.S. registered patient whether or not the patient was actually consulting during the study period. This analysis is concerned only with the activities of the G.P. personnally and not with those undertaken exclusively by the ancillary staff. All his activities even if trivial should be scored whereas tasks completely delegated should not. The writing of a prescription or issue of a sickness certificate are not scored where these form part of the consultation and are absorbed within the Consultation Table (Page 3). The dictation or writing of a referral letter is always scored.

The consultations table is completed during the study and a time schedule for miscellaneous activities is also kept. Results should be summarised appropriately at the end of the study.

																						ENTER FINAL No.
LETTERS – written or dictated																						
To Specialists or Hospitals	1	2	3	4	5	6	7	8	9	10	11	12	13	14	15	16	17	18	19		20	
To Social Workers Housing Depts.etc.	1	2	3	4	5	6	7	8	9	10	11	12	13	14	15	16	17	18	19		20	
Others	1	2	3	4	5	6	7	8	9	10	11	12	13	14	15	16	17	18	19		20	
REPORTS COMPLETED																						
For D.H.S.S.	1	2	3	4	5	6	7	8	9	10	11	12	13	14	15	16	17	18	19		20	
Others	1	2	3	4	5	6	7	8	9	10	11	12	13	14	15	16	17	18	19		20	
REPEAT PRESCRIPTIONS ISSUED																						
	1	2	3	4	5	6	7	8	9	10	11	12	13	14	15	16	17	18	19		20	
	21	22	23	24	25	26	27	28	29	30	31	32	33	34	35	36	37	38	39		40	
	41	42	43	44	45	46	47	48	49	50	51	52	53	54	55	56	57	58	59		60	
	61	62	63	64	65	66	67	68	69	70	71	72	73	74	75	76	77	78	79		80	
	81	82	83	84	85	86	87	88	89	90	91	92	93	94	95	96	97	98	99		100	
INTERVIEWS WITH RELATIVES																						
	1	2	3	4	5	6	7	8	9	10	11	12	13	14	15	16	17	18	19		20	
TELEPHONE CALLS (received or made by Doctor)																						
With Patients or Relatives	1	2	3	4	5	6	7	8	9	10	11	12	13	14	15	16	17	18	19		20	
Hospital Doctors	1	2	3	4	5	6	7	8	9	10	11	12	13	14	15	16	17	18	19		20	
Hospital Other Staff	1	2	3	4	5	6	7	8	9	10	11	12	13	14	15	16	17	18	19		20	
Other Doctors	1	2	3	4	5	6	7	8	9	10	11	12	13	14	15	16	17	18	19		20	
H V SW Midwife etc.	1	2	3	4	5	6	7	8	9	10	11	12	13	14	15	16	17	18	19		20	
Others	1	2	3	4	5	6	7	8	9	10	11	12	13	14	15	16	17	18	19		20	

CONSULTATIONS TABLE

Keep a record of all patients consulting during the two study weeks and enter in the table.

Week 1					Week 2			
CONSULTATIONS A.M.	P.M.	VISITS	CLINICS		CONSULTATIONS A.M.	P.M.	VISITS	CLINICS
				MON				
				TUES				
				WED				
				THUR				
				FRI				
				SAT/SUN				

MISCELLANEOUS ACTIVITY TIME SCHEDULE

Enter the time spent, under each of the appropriate headings, during the study fortnight separating the time involved in travelling.

	ACTIVITY TIME		TRAVELLING TIME	
	hrs.	mins.	hrs.	mins.
Undergraduate Education				
Postgraduate Education (Section 63)				
Postgraduate Education (Non Section 63)				
Tutorials etc. with Trainees				
B.M.A., R.C.G.P., etc. meetings				
Partnership meetings				
Visiting Patients in Hospital				
Other Medical meetings (non remunerative)				
TOTAL				

DATA RETURN SHEET

To obtain a personal and group analysis of your recorded data complete this sheet and return to the leader of your recording group or directly to the Research Unit. (Address on Page 1)

Dr. Name ....

Partnership ....

Address ....

....

Is this the first P.A.A. Data Sheet you have returned to the P.A.A. Unit.

YES ☐   NO ☐

Recording Group (if any) ....

Study Period From .... to .... (enter dates)

Type of Practice (enter one √ on each line)

1 Industrial ☐	Residential ☐	Mixed ☐
2 Urban ☐	Rural ☐	Mixed ☐
3 Dispensing ☐	Non-Dispensing ☐	Mixed ☐

Status of Recorder

Partner ☐   Assistant ☐   Trainee ☐

Practice List Size

Specify Total List Size ....

* Estimated Personal Contribution to Practice

During Study Period .... %

* Examples

Three partners sharing work load equally
Estimated Contribution = 33%

Four partner practice. One on holiday during study and of remaining three one worked part time.
Estimated Contribution = 40%

Single handed doctor. Occasional help with surgeries.
Estimated Contribution = 90%

Trainee. Not possible to estimate.
Estimated Contribution = N.K.

CHOOSING THE TOPIC

Tracer conditions and problems

The range of care given by primary health care teams is so broad that it is not possible to audit everything. Kessner *et al.* (1973) have suggested that topics chosen should either be important in themselves, or broad enough to give an impression of how the practice may be performing in similar activities. Such topics are called *tracers*. Kessner defines the characteristics required for a good tracer in terms of medical conditions, but they can easily be adapted to apply to management problems also.

1. A tracer should have a 'Definite functional impact'. That is to say it must have a noticeable effect on the patients' well being.
2. A tracer should be amenable to change. There is little point in auditing a topic about which nothing can be done.
3. A tracer should be well defined and easy to diagnose.
4. The prevalence rate should be high enough to provide adequate numbers for study.
5. The techniques of management should be well defined.
6. The effect of non-medical factors must be understood. In primary health care these relate mainly to social class: access to doctors may well be determined by social class, just as we know that disease incidence is.

While the definition of tracers gives help in deciding whether any suggested audit topic is suitable, it does not help in deciding which topics the practice wants to take on. Such topics fall into two categories: either the subject is one which has been noticed as a problem by a member of the practice team (examples are given in Chapter 13) or is of such major importance in primary care that it is generally recognized that its management should be audited (such as preventive care or chronic disease management).

Identifying problems

This can be a very good way for a practice team to begin. The problem may have been noticed by anyone on the practice team; receptionists may well see problems in access or management, nurses and doctors are more likely to identify clinical issues. If the practice has a suggestion box the patients may suggest items for review. Problems for audit arising in this way are often small enough to be managed without excessive effort, and are of interest to many team members, so producing a feeling of 'ownership' which both gives stimulus to do the audit and motivation to change in response to it.

The practice does need a system if such audit topics are to be handled efficiently, so that they are not forgotten, and nor does the practice take on too many at once. The practice needs a key person identified, in most cases the practice manager, to hold and maintain a list of topics suggested. Such a list can be available to the partners for discussion, and can also be presented to a practice team meeting so that the practice can decide which problem to tackle. Once such a decision is taken it is likely that a small team will need to be made responsible for the audit.

Choosing the topic for an audit takes the following course:

1. Problem identified by practice team member.
2. Reported to practice manager.
3. The practice manager maintains lists—discussed with partners.
4. Topic for audits selected at practice meeting.
5. Audit team appointed to conduct audit.

Problems identified and handled in this way may well be fairly small projects which can be completed and reported quickly. Some examples are given in Chapter 14. They may also be critical events which can be analysed, or be found to be part of a pattern (Chapter 13). It is very encouraging for a practice to complete some smaller topics and not feel bogged down by embarking on major numerical studies at the outset.

Topics of major importance

Chronic disease management, preventive care, prescribing, and availability are such topics, and examples are provided in Part III. Again, the practice needs to agree on which are to have priority; and who is to form the group responsible for the audit. In choosing priorities there are some points which may influence the practice.

1. *It may help if it is a subject on which data has to be collected anyway.* There are several topics on which the FHSA requires data as part of doctors' terms of service. In particular this applies to childhood immunization, cervical cytology, referrals to hospitals, and use of laboratory services. The figures required by the FHSA may not be very meaningful, and no practice discussion is demanded. But since the data has to be collected anyway the primary health care team may find it useful to collect it in a way which has more significance—for instance, discussing the data and setting targets for the followiing year. In this way external monitoring can be modified into educational audit with little extra effort.
2. *There may be some topics concerning which external help is available.* Thus, preventive procedures, visiting rates or psychotropic prescribing are topics on which the Birmingham RCGP Research Unit has practice activity analysis forms; the local MAAG may have protocols, or may be encouraging audit on a topic common to several practices in the local area; or a local group may

be focusing on a certain subject. There are great advantages in working with others to compare and contrast performance, and it saves a good deal of work if other people's audit protocols can be found which are suitable (so long as the practice is interested in the subject and not doing it just because the data and materials are available).

Structure, process, and outcome

To examine large topics, especially clinical topics, often appears daunting. It can help to break them down into the categories defined by Donabedian (1980), structure, process, and outcome. In starting audit of any topic it is usually most feasible to study structure first, then process, then intermediate outcomes, perhaps over successive audit cycles.

Structure

Structure refers to physical features of the practice; the premises, the availability of staff and their training, clinic times, and so on. It is the least closely related to health outcomes of the three components, but the easiest to study, so usually the best area to start with in an audit.

In an audit of the visual component of child health surveillance, aspects of structure to be assessed might include the presence of health visitors; their education and training in visual screening; the provision of Sheridan Gardner equipment; the evidence of a care plan for vision tests; and the management plan for those failing the test.

Process

Process refers to the activities of the primary health care team in delivering patient care. It is more difficult to observe than structure, but can more often be shown to be related to good outcome.

In the same audit of children's visual development, measures of process would include the proportion of children attending for the prescribed check; the numbers passing and failing; the proportion of those failing the test seen by the ophthalmic services; and the quality of the interaction between the health visitors and the patients.

Outcomes

Outcomes are the results of health care. They are therefore the ideal indicators of care, but the most difficult to measure. Also, by the time outcomes are measured it is too late to make changes to benefit the patients on whom those outcomes were measured.

In the case of children's visual development, outcomes are fairly easy to measure because development takes place rapidly and if deficient should be noted early. Thus an outcome measure would be the number of patients with visual defects found at pre-school medical but previously undiagnosed.

It is unusual to have such clear outcome measures in primary care—numbers are usually too small and outcomes have multifactorial causes and occur after long delay—so *intermediate outcomes* are usually used.

In cardiovascular disease prevention the reduction in risk factors (smoking, blood pressure, lipid levels) is a more meaningful (intermediate) outcome of care than the incidence of myocardial infarction.

ENTERING THE AUDIT CYCLE

The point at which the audit cycle is entered is of no importance (for this reason, no item in the cycle is at the top). The crucial matter is that once the cycle has been entered, the audit exercise must continue until the cycle has been completed at least once.

The theoretically logical starting point is that of setting target standards but that is the most difficult and usually best left until information has been collected. The usual place to enter the cycle is the easiest stage, which is usually that of collecting data, especially if the collection is confined to structure and process. Often it is only with such data to provide evidence of present activity that is it possible to develop plans which are manageable with current resources or targets which are realistic in the light of current achievement.

For instance, in an audit of access to the doctor, the practice may decide to examine how many appointments are offered each week against the number of patients eventually seen; to record at the beginning of each half day how long a patient would have to wait for an appointment with each doctor; and maybe patients' views on accessibility and the relative merits of appointments against wait-your-turn open surgeries. In the light of the findings the practice might plan care (for example, one open surgery each day, the rest appointments), agree criteria for assessment, and set target levels of performance (for example, each doctor should be available within 48 hours, to be achieved in 80 per cent of cases; patients should feel that telephone access is adequate, to be achieved for 90 per cent of patients).

Conversely, the primary health care team might decide to enter the cycle by planning care or implementing change (for example changing the appointment system), then collecting data, making further changes and setting target standards. Observation of practices by MAAG visitors shows that most 'audits' consist of choosing the topic, collecting data, and discussion by the doctors. The elements usually missing are the implementation of change and the setting of target standards (p. 00). Yet, so long as the practice persists in going round a cycle, these two activities will get done, even if not at the outset.

IN SUMMARY

1. Work together as a team.
2. Do what interests you.
3. Keep it small and simple.
4. Look at structure first, then process, then (intermediate) outcome.
5. Enter the cycle at any point, but keep going until all the elements of the cycle have been carried out.

REFERENCES

Baker, R. and Presley, P. (1990). *The practice audit plan*. Severn Faculty RCGP.

Crombie, D. L. and Fleming, D. M. (1988). *Practice activity analysis*. Occasional paper No. 41. RCGP London.

Donabedian, A. (1980). *Exploration in quality assessment and monitoring. Vol 1*. Health Administration Press, Ann Arbor.

Kessner, D. M., Kalk, C. E., and Singer, J. (1973). *Assessing health quality—the case for tracers*. *New England Journal of Medicine*, **288** 189–94.

Lawrence, M. S., Coulter, A., and Jones, L. (1990). *A total audit of preventive procedures in 45 practices caring for 430,000 patients*. *British Medical Journal*, **300**, 1501–3.

5   Setting standards in practice

Neil Johnson

It is only logical to define what it is one is aiming to achieve and set targets for this, before collecting data about performance and trying to interpret it. However, a large number of audits omit this stage altogether. This may not be as surprising as it seems. The language and the definitions involved in standard setting may seem cumbersome and confusing, and while we all tend to resent standards set by others, it is often difficult and time consuming to set our own.

This chapter will explore the concept of 'standard setting' and how this can be achieved in practice.

THE CONCEPT OF SETTING STANDARDS

Chapter 1 described three stages in setting standards.

1. Selecting indicators of care.
2. Developing criteria for those indicators.
3. Setting levels of performance for those criteria.

It is not possible to audit every aspect of care, but in being selective it is important to choose those aspects which are valid indicators of quality. For any topic it is sensible for a practice to consider indicators which cover each of the four main areas of quality, namely, effectiveness, efficiency, equity, and humanity. This may help to avoid a frequent response to the results of an audit 'what you've measured is very interesting but not important to me or my patients'.

A well-defined criterion is one for which it is possible to say for any individual patient whether it has been satisfied or not. Agreeing a criterion does not imply that it has to be achieved in every case, indeed, several criteria can be examined for the same indicator; for example, 'is the fasting blood sugar less than 10 mmol/l?' or 'is it less than 8 mmol/l?' For this reason it is usually possible within and between practices to agree to assess the same criteria, and it is often acceptable to use criteria which have been developed outside the practice.

Conversely, the level of performance is a continuous variable which can lie anywhere between none of the time and all of the time. It is only by attaching a level of performance to a criterion that a standard is set, and by agreeing a target level of performance that a practice sets a target standard. Information from outside may well help to set a reasonable target, but because practice circumstances vary widely and because practices need a dynamic structure for improvement, the target level of performance should be set from within the practice. Whatever the present level of care is found to be, the target standard can be that next bit higher, but should remain within reach and, most of all, it should be right for the practice. This has the benefit of being dynamic, a spur to improvement.

It is also necessary to revise the criteria over time. Minimum criteria, even though they may be achieved all the time, only represent a minimum standard of care. This of course is what results from setting minimum standards of care; it establishes a threshold above which it is necessary to pass to avoid censure, but in the process aspirations may be lowered to that level. If, however, a practice aspires to criteria which are more difficult to achieve, it will be aspiring to higher standards of overall care, and may be achieving them, even though the criteria may not be achieved all the time.

Separating criteria from levels of performance also clarifies what the confusion and resistance over standards may be due to. For example, in the 1990 contract for general practice, target payments were introduced if more than 80 per cent of women aged 35–64 had had an adequate cervical smear within the last 5.5 years. Many practices complained that this was unfair; but some argued that the implied criterion that all women should have a cervical smear was wrong, and that account should be taken of nuns, virgins, and patients who chose to say no, while others argued that the level of performance required was unattainable in many practice circumstances.

In conclusion, when a practice is setting its standards it should establish a list of criteria that are agreed by the practice, but may or may not have come from other sources, together with a target level of performance for each criterion which reflects the circumstances and the progress that that practice is making.

DEVELOPING CRITERIA

As in any other form of assessment the criteria used should be both valid and reliable. A valid criterion is one that has a demonstrable or at least agreed relationship to the quality and outcome of care. A further measure of validity is the extent to which the criterion is agreed by those who will be involved in the audit. A reliable criterion is one whose achievement can either be measured or judged in such a way that the degree of agreement between two observers, or the same observer on two separate occasions, as to whether the criterion had or had not been achieved would be substantially greater than would occur by chance. It is difficult to do this unless a criterion is explicitly stated. Useful criteria should be:

1. Related to aspects of quality, namely, effectiveness, efficiency, equity, and humanity.

2. Related to desirable outcomes.
3. Explicit. It should be possible to write down the criteria in a clear concise fashion for discussion and review.
4. Acceptable. The criteria should be acceptable to all members of the team whose care is going to be assessed.
5. Assessable. It should be possible to measure the degree of achievement of each criterion.

There are a number of ways of getting information which help to agree a set of criteria.

Information from clinical trials

Ideally, a criterion is a favourable outcome of care or an item in the structure or process of care which has been demonstrated to result in favourable outcomes in clinical trials. A literature search or a good review article may well produce some such criteria, for example, the control of high blood pressure leading to reduced risk of stroke (Medical Research Council Working Party 1985); organized diabetic care and a reduction in hospital admissions (Farmer and Coulter 1990); and negotiation in consultations and subsequent compliance with medication and life-style advice (Carr 1990). Caution is sometimes necessary in applying research findings derived from a clinical trial to a different population of patients in everyday general practice, but this is probably less of a danger than our frequent failure to apply existing knowledge in practice.

Validated professional opinion

There are two major studies which have produced criteria via a two stage process. Grol (1990) and his colleagues in the Netherlands established an expert panel to produce draft criteria which they then offered to a reference panel of practising doctors for comment. They showed that their criteria were acceptable and that their use brought about change in the behaviour of doctors. However there were problems. First, for each clinical topic they offered a great number of criteria and it is difficult to separate out which might be most useful to us. Secondly, although research has demonstrated their use in affecting doctors' behaviour, the scientific basis for any single criterion was not stated. Thirdly, the criteria for Dutch doctors cannot necessarily be directly related to a practice in the UK.

The second group studying in this field does come from the UK. The North of England Study (1990) considered the effect of using clinical guidelines on the outcome for care. They showed that involvement in the process of developing the guidelines resulted in both an improvement in doctors' clinical performance and in the long-term outcome for patients. These results should be very encouraging to us, but again there are problems. First, the participants produced sets of clinical guidelines, for example an algorithm, rather than criteria; and secondly, like the Dutch group, the scientific basis for their guidelines is not stated, so the clinical validity is not clear.

Because of these difficulties it may not be possible simply to borrow criteria from these studies, but they do at least show that developing and adopting guidelines can make a difference to the quality of care.

Expert opinion

Expert opinion is often available to practices either from local specialists or from published review articles.

Sometimes these reviews are based on a consensus of opinion of those active in the relevant field (for example, the British Thoracic Society 1990). These are usually published in the form of guidelines for care and it may be necessary to take such guidelines and develop criteria from them. This may be helpful as it takes advantage of the expertise as well as saving time, but it is necessary to determine whether the guidelines are suitable for use in one's own practice. The questions that may need to be answered include:

1. What is the basis of the guidelines? Are they based on published research, consensus, individual opinion, or audit undertaken in a group of practices? This gives some idea of their clinical validity.
2. Do the guidelines seem realistic? If they are to be useful then it must be possible to follow them in everyday practice.
3. Is the setting similar to your own?
4. Can precise criteria be developed from the guidelines?

Practice based criteria

Sometimes there is little published or outside opinion to guide the practice and it may be necessary for a practice to develop their criteria entirely 'in house'. It can take a lot of time and effort to ensure that they are valid, but one method of short cutting this is to use the methodology described by Grol by requesting a single member or subgroup of the team to produce drafts of criteria for presentation back to their colleagues. This consultation must be carried out during the production of the criteria, or else the rest of the team may not feel any ownership and so will be less likely to adhere to the criteria when they are finally produced. One method that may be helpful in reducing some of the time involved is to circulate the proposed criteria to all members of the team and invite them to agree or disagree, and then to focus discussion time on the areas of disagreement. Areas of disagreement may also lead to further consultation of the literature or expert opinion.

SETTING THE LEVEL OF PERFORMANCE

The final stage in setting standards is to set the target level of performance. It was argued earlier that it is crucial that this should be set from within the practice. How do we decide what is an appropriate target level? There are three ways of getting information on what is likely to be appropriate. First, published research may well show the level to which a criterion is likely to be performed. For instance, Grol shows that even amongst those who supported the development of criteria, only 30–70 per cent of the agreed criteria were achieved.

Secondly, the experience of other groups or neighbouring practices can give an estimate of the likely level of performance that could be attained. This information may also come from published studies of audits, from local audit groups, or more formally through the MAAGs. The Birmingham Research Unit of the RCGP (1977) in their Practice Activity Analysis programme, collected data from participating practices on aspects of their activity and provided feedback to individual practices of their performance compared with the distribution of performance in all the practices participating in the study. This allowed practices to know where they stood in relationship to their colleagues.

Finally, when attempting to set an appropriate target level of performance, it is worth looking at the level that has already been achieved and considering whether it is adequate and how much realistic scope there is for improvement. Clearly, if one is assessing a topic on which other practices' data are available, then combining what is known about one's own performance with what is known about others' performance should help in the choice of a target level of performance that is both appropriate for one's own group and also in line with others.

GUIDELINES AND PROTOCOLS

So far in this chapter we have seen how, by selecting criteria and setting target levels of performance, a practice can set itself targets for any topic of care. But the practice will also need to agree a plan for the management and delivery of that care. The care plan for any topic, together with the arrangements for auditing that care, constitute a protocol: ideally a written document available to any member of the team. Exactly the same processes are involved in agreeing protocols as were involved in agreeing target standards. They can be based on published guidelines available from a variety of sources, but such guidelines' validity, acceptability, and applicability in practice all need to be questioned. As any protocol will be describing the precise way in which the practice intends to work the final version will almost always need to be produced 'in house'.

Just as external criteria could be used as a basis for developing practice target standards, so external guidelines can be helpful as a basis for practice protocols which need to be agreed by the professionals involved in care.

External	Practice agreed
Criteria $\longrightarrow$	Target standards
Guidelines $\longrightarrow$	Protocols

Again, an individual or subgroup may produce a draft protocol, but the process for obtaining agreement and commitment cannot be ·omitted. It is important that protocols should not become too detailed or too idealistic, or this may result in them being ignored. It is better to begin with simple protocols which are used and develop them later if greater rigour is felt desirable.

CONCLUSION

The emphasis of this chapter has been an approach to setting standards which is explicit, flexible, openly discussed, and agreed. There is a danger that this may make undertaking audit seem more daunting, but the investment of time and thought at the outset will undoubtedly pay great dividends when the time comes to assess the value of the results.

REFERENCES

The Birmingham Research Unit of the Royal College of General Practitioners. (1977). Self evaluation in general practice. *Journal of the Royal College of General Practitioners*, **27**, 265–70.

British Thoracic Society. (1990). Guidelines for the management of asthma in adults. *British Medical Journal*, **301**, 651–3, 797–800.

Carr, A. (1990). Compliance with medical advice. *British Journal of General Practice*, **40**, 358–440.

Farmer, A. and Coulter, A. (1990). Organisation of care for diabetic patients in general practice: influence on hospital admission. *British Journal of General Practice*, **40**, 56–8.

Grol, R. (1990). National standard setting for quality of care in general practice: attitudes of general practitioners and response to a set of standards. *British Journal of General Practice*, **40**, 361–4.

Health Departments of Great Britain. (1989). General Practice in the National Health Service: The 1990 Contract. London.

Medical Research Council Working Party. (1985). MRC trial of treatment of mild hypertension: principal results. *British Medical Journal*, **291**, 97–104.

North of England Study of Standards and Performance in General Practice. (1990). Final Report: Volume 1—Setting Clinical Standards within small groups. Report 40. Health Care Research Unit, Newcastle upon Tyne.

6 Collecting and analysing data

David Mant and Patricia Yudkin

INTRODUCTION

Objective

All of the audits described in other chapters of this book require some collection and analysis of data. These tasks need special skills which are simple and well worth acquiring. They will not only save energy and resources, but will mean that the information obtained from reviewing the data is more likely to be an accurate reflection of what is happening in practice.

Avoiding problems

Collecting and analysing data is a common cause of problems. It tends to generate large amounts of paper covered with figures which never quite add up. A number of simple skills can make things simpler, in particular knowing how to:

(1) identify patients;
(2) take samples;
(3) collect data;
(4) analyse data;
(5) make comparisons.

This chapter will consider these skills in practical terms, without going into exhaustive detail. Readers who wish to know more should seek local advice and consult the further reading recommended at the end of the chapter.

IDENTIFYING PATIENTS: ISSUES

Rates

Most audits involve the calculation of rates. The number of times an event has happened must be related to the number of times it could have happened—and this involves identifying not only the patients in whom it did happen, but also those in whom it could have happened. A rate is 'did happen'—the numerator—divided by 'could have happened'—the denominator.

The identification of the group of patients or events forming the denominator is the most important, and sometimes the most difficult, aspect of audit. Most audits have as their denominator a group of patients identified because of a certain characteristic — they may have a specific illness, lie in a certain age/sex group, or be eligible for certain types of care. Some audits are based on events rather than patients — for example, a review of waiting times in the health centre might be based on a certain block of appointments.

Whether in producing the numerator or denominator, if the procedure for identifying the group of patients or events on which the audit is to be based is not specific or complete enough this will lead to bias and any results are likely to be misleading.

Clinical bias

Choosing the group of patients to whom an event 'could happen' is an art of good auditing. For instance, in reviewing patients referred for hysterectomy, the size of the combined doctors' list could be used as the denominator. But patients referred for hysterectomy are usually female and aged 35–60 years, so the number of female patients in that age band would be a better denominator. However, that masks the fact that a female doctor may be seeing more women than a male doctor in a combined list practice, so it may be necessary to identify a separate denominator for each partner, using the number of women aged 35–60 years seen in the relevant time period. Unless the denominator is chosen to reflect the clinical activity, the results will be misleading.

Definitions and coding

Ascertainment will be incomplete if a decision is taken to audit a particular clinical topic without deciding in advance how to define it. This means agreeing within a practice which specific diagnosis will be used, and whether the cases will be labelled in terms of presenting symptoms or presumptive diagnosis.

It should be particularly simple for computerized practices to produce lists of patients by clinical categories. But, although at least one general practice coding system (Read) is available which is almost exhaustive in its possibilities, it is still very difficult to achieve the consistency of coding diagnoses which makes the identification of patient groups straightforward.

For example, in reviewing the management of sore throats the practice may agree to enter 'sore throat' for all cases, or several entries may be allowed, such as sore throat, tonsillitis, pharyngitis, or laryngitis. If any descriptions are used and not included in a search, then ascertainment will be incomplete and the sample may be biased. For instance, cases entered as 'tonsillitis' are likely to be more severe than those entered as 'sore throat', so an analysis based on sore throat entries will be biased towards the milder cases.

Response bias

It is tempting to conduct audits on patients who attend, or to carry out analysis on questionnaires from people who reply. But unless a high proportion of the eligible population attend for the service or return the questionnaire, then those who do are unlikely to be a representative sample. Attenders and responders tend to be healthier, of higher social class, more compliant with management, and non-smokers. It is generally felt that a response rate of about 80 per cent is necessary for a sample to be acceptable as representative.

Worst first bias

The 'worst first bias' results from the fact that serious problems are more likely to be recorded than less serious ones. This bias was first described in the context of prevention, when it was noted that practices with low recording rates for smoking habit identified mainly heavy smokers. It is also true for chronic disease registration: the average severity is likely to be inversely proportional to the ascertainment rate. A comparative audit of outcome in patients identified from chronic disease registers will therefore produce very different results in practices with high and low registration rates, simply because practices with the low rates are likely to be auditing less healthy patients. The solution to this bias is to use several sources to maximize the number of patients identified, or for the practice to concentrate on keeping a complete disease register for some time before auditing.

Source bias

Patients are often identified from some characteristic in the medical record. But if the characteristic on which the identification is based is correlated with an aspect of the care being audited then results can again be misleading.

For example, an audit of patients with hypothyroidism could be done using as the denominator patients who order repeat prescriptions. But those currently taking treatment exclude those who have defaulted from care or who have been lost to follow-up: an audit of such patients will be falsely reassuring. Attendance at a clinic is another characteristic which could be used to identify patients. But again, this method will overestimate the proportion of patients under medical review.

Problems of measurement

Awareness of measurement error is important, in that a group of patients is often identified on the basis of a threshold level: for example those with diastolic blood pressure greater than 95 mmHg or with cholesterol level greater than 6.5 mmol/l. But in all measurement there is error, and it is often larger than expected.

For example, blood cholesterol levels vary between winter and summer, and in an individual from day to day. Measurements on an individual should therefore be repeated to give that person's average value. Laboratory measurement is subject to error, and two measurements made on the same blood sample would be expected to produce somewhat different results.

The coefficient of variation is a measure of the repeatability of laboratory results. Figure 6.1 relates the actual value of cholesterol in a blood sample (6.2 mmol/l) to the values that might be reported by different laboratories. For example, a laboratory working with a 5 per cent coefficient of variation (generally considered to be an acceptable level) would have a 5 per cent chance of reporting the cholesterol level in the blood sample as high as 6.8 mmol/l or as low as 5.6 mmol/l. Because of this natural variation and measurement imprecision it is important to make repeated measurements before assigning a patient to a category on the basis of measurement.

IDENTIFYING PATIENTS: SOURCES

Traditional sources

There are three traditional sources for the identification of patients and events for audit which are available to virtually all practices. These are patients' diagnostic histories, the repeat prescribing register, and the appointment list. The accessibility of these sources depends very much on whether they are computerized. Fully computerized practices can rapidly use all three sources to generate accurate denominators for almost any audit. A combination of the medical histories and the repeat prescribing list can be used to identify groups with specific diseases. A combination of the medical record and the appointment list can be used to generate a denominator based on age specific, or even disease specific episodes. The same data are available to practices with entirely manual recording systems, but collating the data is much harder work and the production of morbidity related denominators may be impossible unless careful disease registers have been maintained.

New sources

Recent changes in contractual arrangements with FHSAs have been a major source of irritation to general practitioners, but they have also produced new sources of data. General practitioners are expected to keep full records of investigations, referrals, and preventive activities. These data are numerators for the FHSA, which uses the practice list as denominator when reviewing the practice's activity. But they have great potential for use by the practice as denominators, because they indicate patients with particular problems or illnesses.

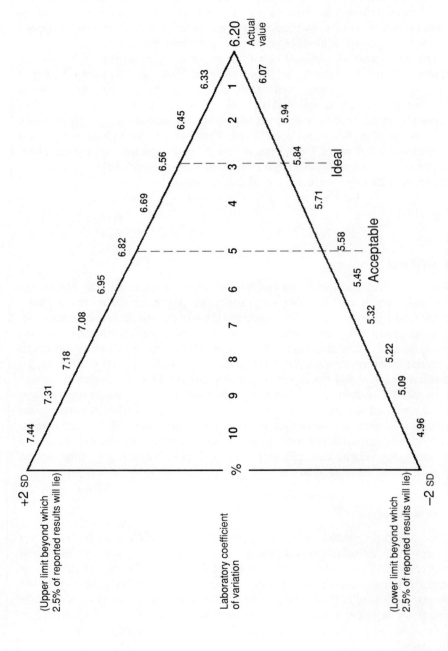

Fig. 6.1 Laboratory analytical imprecision and cholesterol measurement.

The register of investigations is available for examining administrative issues, such as lost specimens, or clinical issues, such as rates of abnormality. The referral register is a good starting point, not only for reviewing the care at hospital but the quality of follow-up at the practice. In prevention, the cervical cytology register contains information about hysterectomy; and the health promotion register information about blood pressure, obesity, and smoking.

Special sources

A number of audits described in this book mention the need to collect data which are not routinely available. For instance, in Chapter 15 on access, a special collecting form is suggested which would be completed solely for the purpose of conducting the audit. Similar special data collection would be necessary to assess patient views on the outcomes of care, or to conduct administrative audits, such as the ease of telephone access. However, it is not necessary to design the collection forms anew on every occasion. It is likely that such an audit has been carried out in at least one other practice and a telephone call to the local MAAG may be very rewarding.

One of the more interesting forms of audit is concerned with 'critical incidents' in practice (Chapter 13). This is an extension of the traditional morbidity conference held in teaching hospitals, and some practices already conduct such audits informally in practice meetings. It is possible to audit deaths, hospitalizations, doctor perceived problems, or any other series of adverse or unexpected events of interest to the practice. The best way to collect cases is probably by doctor held diaries. Hospital admission or discharge notifications and death notifications are other good sources.

A rather neglected means of identifying a group of patients for audit is through hospital recorded data on morbidity and clinical activity. Hospital computers now record routinely the doctor or practice with which each hospitalized patient is registered. The quality of coding and the ready availability of data varies greatly from District to District, but it is well worth enquiry to the Region or District Information Manager to see exactly what is available. Out-patient and pathology/X-ray databases are being developed.

TAKING SAMPLES

A number of chapters recommend collecting audit information by sampling. Sampling saves time and energy, and often allows a reasonable estimate to be made without examining every set of notes or consulting every patient. However, it is not entirely straightforward and there are a number of issues to be considered before taking the plunge.

Simple and systematic sampling

The traditional method of sampling (called simple random sampling) is by the use of random number tables. This usually produces a good representative sample, but it is time consuming and rather cumbersome. For example, to draw a 5 per cent sample of medical records, every patient's record is assigned a number, and then random number tables are used to select records until a 5 per cent sample has been chosen.

The method of choice in general practice is systematic sampling. This means arranging the items to be audited in sequence and sampling every *n*th item in a predetermined pattern. In general, systematic sampling of this kind is reasonably bias free. For example, to draw a 5 per cent sample of medical records you could list the patients alphabetically and draw every 20th record.

Systematic sampling from medical record stacks suffers from two potential sources of bias. First, the records of 'active' patients may not be in the record stack but out for use in and around the surgery. The records which are most likely to be in the stack are those of 'ghosts' (patients who are still on the register but who have died or gone away). If the proportion of ghosts and notes missing from the stack at any one time is small, the potential for serious bias is similarly small. If not, then sampling from an alternative source, such as an age/sex register would be preferable—and this is increasingly straightforward since most computerized practices can print out such a list.

The second potential bias is due to the fact that medical records are not filed in random order. Families, or even entire nationalities, may occur together if the records are filed in alphabetical order. If the records are filed by street name then patients from similar socio-economic and cultural groups will be adjacent. In order to avoid serious bias it is important that the sample is drawn from the entire stack and not from one particular part of it.

Sample size

When it is decided to use a sample then the question always arises 'How many records must I examine—or patients must I interview—to obtain adequate data on which to base my audit?'.

Suppose, for example, that you want to discover the percentage of patients on treatment for hypertension who have had a blood pressure taken in the last year. In general, the larger the sample, the closer the sample result will be to the 'correct' or 'population' percentage—that is, the value that would have been obtained by auditing *all* the records. But because each sample will include a different assortment of patients, even a large sample may occasionally produce a misleading result, and how well a particular sample represents *all* patients can never be completely certain. It is possible only to make statements such as: 'There is a probability of 95 per cent (i.e. it is extremely likely) that the sample result is not more than 5 per cent (or 2.5 per cent or 1 per cent) different from the correct value'. The maximum difference from the correct (population) value could be termed the error of the sample result. This error will tend to be smaller with bigger samples.

This means that one factor in determining sample size is the size of the error that can be tolerated. But there are two additional factors that affect the required sample size: the number of patients being audited (with more patients the sample needs to be bigger, although a smaller proportion of the total) and, perhaps surprisingly, the actual percentage of patients satisfying the criterion in question (the closer this value to 50 per cent the bigger the sample needed).

In planning the sample size needed for an audit the following factors must therefore be considered.

1. What is the size of the possible error that can be tolerated?

   This is essentially a matter of judgement, but it will depend to some extent on the expected result. For example, in an audit of cervical cytology it might be expected that about 80 per cent of women aged between 30 and 65 years would have had a cervical smear (and 20 per cent would not). A practice might be satisfied to estimate these percentages to within 5 per cent of their true value. But in an audit of child immunization, perhaps 90 per cent of children would have been immunized and only 10 per cent would not. In this case the possible error that could be tolerated might be reduced to 2.5 per cent.

2. How many patients are being audited?

   The relevant number will not usually be the entire practice list, but rather the number of patients eligible to meet the criterion in question. For example, women aged between 35 and 64 years, or children aged less than 5 years, (see rates, p. 56).

3. What is the expected answer?

   It may appear illogical to have to know the results of the audit in order to calculate the sample size needed to carry it out, but it is the case that the error attached to a percentage figure derived from a sample depends partly on the actual percentage itself. In planning sample size then, an estimate has to be made of this percentage.

   Table 6.1 gives the sample sizes needed in different circumstances. For example, suppose that after a screening programme a practice wanted to find out how many of its female patients aged between 50 and 64 years had accepted a mammogram. Assume that the practice had 1000 women in this age group, and that the best a priori guess was that about 70 per cent would meet this criterion. Table 6.1a shows that to have a 95 per cent probability

Table 6.1 *Size of sample required for 95 per cent probability that the true result lies within 5 per cent or 2.5 per cent of the estimate*

(a) For accuracy of estimate ±5 per cent

| Number in group being audited | \<div>Best guess of likely result\</div> | | | | |
	10 or 90%	20 or 80%	30 or 70%	40 or 60%	50%
50	35	40	40	45	45
100	60	70	80	80	80
250	90	120	140	150	150
500	110	170	200	210	220
1000	120	200	240	270	280
3000	130	230	290	330	340
5000	140	230	300	340	360

(b) For accuracy of estimate ±2.5 per cent

| Number in group being audited | Best guess of likely result | | | | |
	10 or 90%	20 or 80%	30 or 70%	40 or 60%	50%
50	45	50	50	50	50
100	85	90	90	95	95
250	170	200	210	210	220
500	260	330	360	370	380
1000	360	500	560	600	610
3000	470	740	900	990	1020
5000	500	820	1030	1140	1180

of estimating the percentage to within 5 per cent of the correct value, a sample of 240 would be needed. To make an estimate that would very probably be within 2.5 per cent of the correct value, a larger sample, of 560, would be required.

Note that (as mentioned above) the largest sample would be needed when the a priori guess of the result is 50 per cent. There are two reasons why opting for this largest sample may be the best strategy. First, it may simply not be possible to make a realistic guess of the result, especially with a topic that has not been audited before in the practice. Secondly, many general practice audits involve looking at various criteria in one sample, and the maximum sample size would cover all eventualities.

Readers who prefer a graphical presentation can use Fig. 6.2 to read off the largest required size of sample to provide a result that has 95 per cent probability of being within 5 per cent of the true result.

The formula on which these sample size calculations were based is given in the Appendix to this chapter. This will allow sample sizes to be calculated for circumstances not covered by the tables or figure.

COLLECTING DATA

Keeping good records

If patient records are to be used for audit, the data must have been regularly recorded in the first place, and in a way in which it can be quickly and easily extracted. Mant and Tulloch (1987) showed a large deficit in the recording of major diagnoses in general practice records, compared with hospital discharge data, and Coulter *et al.* (1992) had to employ a full time research assistant to extract information from general practitioners' notes about events before and after a hospital referral.

Both problems are reduced by a flow card (manual records), or a dedicated screen or template (computerized records). An example of a flow card for asthma management is shown on p. 131. Such flow cards and screens combine several benefits:

1. They act as prompts for checks which have been omitted or are overdue.
2. They assemble data into one place, so that decisions can be made on multi-factorial risk.
3. The need to enter data in a predetermined way reduces the risk of different primary health care team members using different criteria for diagnosis, management, and recording.
4. They make data extraction quicker, by providing the data in an organized and summarized way.

Extracting data from the records

Using manual systems, the most common way of extracting data from patient records is to draw up a list of the indicators to be examined and then go through each record in turn, recording *either* the indicator (for example, the diastolic blood pressure) or whether a criterion for that indicator has been satisfied (for example, was the diastolic blood pressure less than 90 mmHg?). Examples of such lists are shown on p. 126 for diabetes, and p. 156 for termination of

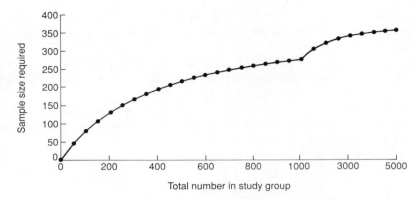

Fig. 6.2 Graph showing the largest sample size required for 95 per cent probability of the true result lying within 5 per cent of the estimate, for varying size of study group.

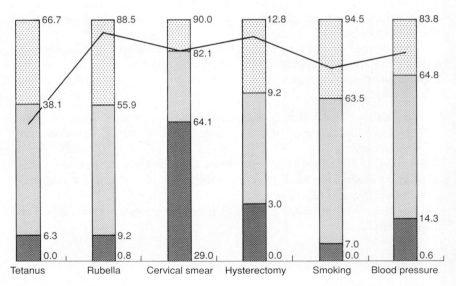

Fig. 6.3 One practice's results superimposed on a histogram derived from 45 other practices' data. The top of each column is the highest figure recorded by any practice, the bottom the lowest. The shading changes at the 20th and 80th centiles. These examples show the percentage of at risk patients recorded immune to tetanus, immune to rubella, with adequate cervical cytology, having had a hysterectomy, with smoking status known, and with blood pressure recorded in the last five years.

pregnancy. The development of such lists is best done by a sub-group of the practice team, with data extraction and summarizing being delegated to a member of the team.

Some FHSAs offer a service, sometimes known as 'Rent-an-audit' (Gray *et al.* 1987), by which audit clerks can be hired by a practice to come and extract data, often according to FHSA approved criteria. But this procedure is liable to reduce the ownership and commitment of the practice, so a working method within the practice team is preferable.

Sometimes data merely need to be collected routinely and aggregated on to a summary chart. Examples would be the ongoing collections of consultations or visits so that work rate can be calculated; or the monitoring of doctors' prescriptions to check compliance with a formulary (Chapter 12).

Data extraction is clearly most efficiently done by computers. The search criteria take the place of the criteria list used manually, and the computer search removes the need for the routine work of extracting and examining records. Such data extraction depends on the data having been entered regularly, and entered in a coded or numeric form that is easy for the computer to search — it is more difficult to search data entered in free text.

Two developments are making computerized data extraction even simpler. First, report generators offer the facility to record a search and rerun it again at any chosen time in the future. In this way, practices can develop a library of searches and then run them, often overnight at regular intervals, to monitor change. Secondly, audit programs can be written externally and provided for practices who can send their results on floppy disk for central analysis. Practices then receive their own results in comparison with all other participating practices. (An example providing data for practices using VAMP computers is shown in Fig. 6.3).

Data very useful in undertaking audit are also collected by bodies external to practices. FHSAs collect a great deal on practice structure (such as the number of type of doctors and staff), administrative process (such as night visits and clinics), and even some outcomes (such as cytology and immunization figures). PACT is available from the national prescription pricing bureau (Chapter 12). All these data are available and require no collection effort on the part of the practice.

However, it has to be emphasized, particularly now that data extraction is becoming so much easier and often need not involve medical staff at all, that data collection is not audit. It is only the first stage in an audit. To be valuable it is necessary to evaluate the data, plan care on the basis of that evaluation, and set new targets.

Monitoring activity using a pro forma

Not all data can be extracted from records retrospectively, because the required information may not have been routinely and regularly collected. In this case, data have to be collected prospectively, usually by the use of a special form to ensure that required data are collected for the duration of the study.

A study of access and availability is an example (Chapter 15) where the practice wishes to assess its availability, but the effort of recording it does not justify continuous record keeping—so a form is used to enable the availability to be monitored from time to time. Patients' waiting times in surgery would be a further example whereby doctors could record the time at which a patient entered the consulting room and this could be analysed in conjunction with the booked time.

The development of pro formas is not easy. It is necessary to:

(1) obtain information which is relevant;
(2) define terms which are unambiguous;
(3) ensure that the information required is not too extensive;
(4) devise a system so that recording is reliable;
(5) achieve data which are not too complicated to analyse.

When developing a pro forma it is necessary to show it to several other members of the team to ensure that it is intelligible, and to receive as much constructive criticism as possible. It then helps to pilot the study on a small sample: and when the pro forma is used in the practice it must be evaluated in conjunction with the findings, to examine in what way it can be improved before the data collection is repeated. Pro formas have been developed for many topics, for example availability (Chapter 15) or management of sore throat (Chapter 14). A phone call to the local MAAG may enable practices to use or adapt others' pro formas rather than starting from the beginning.

Collecting data by questionnaire or interview

It is often necessary to obtain information from patients, either to elicit their views, or to find out something about their health status or history. This can be done by questionnaire, which is relatively quick and cheap but may provide poor response rates and gives no opportunity for explaining ambiguities; or it can be done by interview, which usually provides more reliable data but at greatly increased cost.

For either purpose a data collection form will be required, and the design of such forms may produce inaccurate or inadequate data unless certain rules are adhered to. Such design is considered in Chapter 16 'Audit of patients' views'; readers wishing a more extensive treatment of the subject should consult Wilkin *et al.* (1992).

ANALYSING THE DATA

Good audits should require minimal analysis. Simple, well thought out questions usually provide simple answers. The need for complex analysis often suggests insufficient thought went into the initial design. Nevertheless, even the most simple audit requires manipulation, such as adding up and calculation of rates.

Manual analysis

It is not necessary to analyse small data sets by computer. It is just as easy to use a calculator. Modern calculators have a number of functions which makes the calculation of rates and percentages very straightforward. However, to go beyond this without using a computer should be avoided if possible. There are three types of software package which may be helpful—spreadsheets, databases, and analytical software.

Spreadsheets

The most widely available and easy to use software is a spreadsheet. It provides a balance sheet of rows and columns and will not only add up the rows and columns (without making any mistakes), but will also manipulate any of the rows and columns in any way you like. For example, it will allow you to divide one column by another, thus calculating rates in seconds. Some spreadsheets are more sophisticated and will calculate means, medians, etc, but they are generally not as powerful for this sort of operation as database software.

Database software

Most of the commercial general practice systems work by creating a database and providing software to interrogate that database. Groups of patients can be identified and subdivided according to common characteristics. For example, one could list all patients with diabetes or all patients taking oral contraceptives, and then subdivide them by characteristics such as age and smoking status. In short, it is possible to relate any item on a database to any other. However, in practice, the software used by most commercial general practice systems is much less flexible for these tasks than independent database software.

Simple database software is most impressive. A package such as dBase allows the relatively inexperienced user to set up screens for data entry; to sort lists and correlate the data items in any combination; and to perform more sophisticated analyses by simple programming. The latest version of dBase and similar packages are very 'user friendly' and a number of general practitioners have become very enthusiastic and adept in their use.

Analytical software

The sort of multi-purpose analytical programs which a few years ago were available only on large mainframe computers are now readily available on microcomputers. They are also 'user friendly' and the instructions appear on the screens as 'menus'. They have two major advantages over databases. First, they perform much more sophisticated analyses very quickly, providing cross tabulations and statistics on most practice audits in a matter of seconds. Secondly, it is possible to prepare the data in the practice using a simple word processing package, such as Wordstar, and then to read the data into the analytical package.

It is relatively easy to learn to use an analytical package. Although some are quite expensive to buy, one (EPI-INFO) is now available free as public domain software. There is no doubt that an audit from a large practice would be best analysed using such software. The easiest way to achieve this for most practices would be to encode the data in the practice using word processing or database software and then to analyse the data elsewhere. Analytical software, including EPI-INFO, will certainly be available in the university departments and possibly in FHSAs. These departments may also help with software programs which perform specific analyses.

Practices needing guidance on software for data collection and analysis should consult their local university department; or their MAAG may be able to point them in the right direction.

MAKING COMPARISONS

The ultimate objective of audit is to change clinical practice to improve the quality of care. This implies that comparisons must be made, perhaps between practices, or between different times in the same practice. In making comparisons, several quite different problems must be considered.

Comparing results from samples

The first problem relates to the fact that the audit may have been based on a sample. As we have seen, any sample result includes a possible error, and this has to be taken into account when making the comparison. Suppose, for example, that an audit of cervical cytology, based on a sample of women aged 35–64 years, showed that 78 per cent (±5 per cent) had had a cervical smear. When the audit was repeated two years later, the result was 84 per cent (±5 per cent). Does this show a real improvement in practice? Or is the apparent increase in the percentage receiving a cervical smear a chance result due to the possible error inherent in the sample estimate?

The error attached to the *difference* between two sample results is a combination—but not a simple sum—of the separate errors attached to each sample result. If the separate errors are equal, and of size δ, the error attached to the difference between sample results is $\sqrt{2} \times \delta$. For example, if each of these errors is ±5 per cent, as in the above example, the error attached to the difference will be $\sqrt{2} \times 5$; i.e. about 7 per cent. The difference between the two cervical smear rates is therefore 6 per cent ± 7 per cent; i.e. had all the records been audited, there is a 95 per cent probability that the difference in smear rates would have been between −1 per cent and 13 per cent. Since this range includes zero, the results are consistent with no real change in the percentage of women screened, but they are also consistent with a substantial increase in this percentage.

A general formula for calculating the error attached to the difference between sample results is given in the Appendix.

Taking the subject of the audit into account

A second problem relates to the activity being audited. Some activities are fully under the control of the practice, others are influenced by factors beyond the general practitioner's control. As an example of the first type, suppose that a practice carried out an audit of immunization against measles in children aged under 5 years, and that this audit was repeated the following year. In the first year the result was 88 per cent and in the second year 92 per cent (assume that full audits had been made, so that there was no problem of sampling error). The audit results would represent a real increase in the percentage of children immunized in the practice. The causes of this improvement could be investigated; they might include an improvement in practice record-keeping, increased efficiency by the practice doctors, or more co-operative parents. In this example, the number of children eligible to be immunized would be known, and the process of immunization would be largely under the general practitioners' control.

Now imagine a different audit—this time of the rate of referrals to gynaecology clinics of women aged 35–74 years. Again, suppose that a full audit had been taken, that there were 4000 women in the age band and that 22 per 1000 were referred in the first year and 28 per 1000 in the second. This represents a real increase in gynaecology referrals, but an important difference from the previous example is that in this case the practice was responding to clinical events (the presentation of particular symptoms in women of a given age) which occur in a quite unpredictable way. The observed increase in referrals is more likely to have resulted from this random fluctuation in the occurrence of disease than from any change in referral behaviour by the general practitioners in the practice.

To assess the meaning of changes in rates of clinical events such as referrals, it is therefore helpful to know how much variation in such rates could have been expected to occur by chance. Table 6.2 (Coulter *et al.* 1991) gives the expected size of this random variation. The table gives the range of variation that would be expected by chance for each average referral rate shown in the left hand column. Of course the true average is not known, but for any practice or individual doctor the best estimate would be the average over several recent years; returning to the example of gynaecology referrals the best guess over the

Table 6.2 *Expected random variation in referral rates based on 95 per cent confidence limits (from Coulter* et al. *1991)* — see text for explanation on use

Average referral rate/1000 patients/year	Number of patients on practice list, or in relevant age/sex group						
	2000	4000	6000	8000	10000	12000	16000
1	2	1	1	1	1	1	1
3	3	2	2	1	1	1	1
5	3	3	2	2	1	1	1
10	5	3	3	2	2	2	2
15	6	4	3	3	3	3	2
20	6	4	4	3	3	3	2
25	7	5	4	4	3	3	2
30	8	5	4	4	3	3	3
40	9	6	5	4	4	4	3
50	10	7	6	5	4	4	3
60	11	8	7	5	5	4	4
70	12	8	7	6	5	5	4
80	13	9	7	6	6	5	4
90	13	9	8	7	6	5	5
100	14	10	8	7	6	6	5
120	15	11	9	8	7	6	5
140	17	12	10	8	7	7	6
160	18	13	10	9	8	7	6
180	19	13	11	9	8	8	7
200	20	14	11	10	9	8	7
220	21	15	12	10	9	8	7
240	22	15	12	11	10	9	8

two years would be 25 per 1000. Table 6.2 shows that with 4000 patients a variation in referral rates of 5 per 1000 would be expected. This would mean referral rates of between 20 and 30 per 1000. The practice rates of 22 and 28 are well within the expected range of random fluctuation, and do not mean that referral behaviour has changed.

Age specific data and age/sex standardization

A further problem in making comparisons, particularly between practices, is that health and medical activity are strongly dependent on the patients' age and sex. So a practice looking after undergraduates in Oxford would expect a very different work pattern from a practice caring for many retired elderly in Bournemouth.

There are two ways of overcoming this problem. One is to compare the management of patients in specific age/sex bands: for instance, both practices would only look at inhaler prescription rates for patients aged 30—64 years. The second is to standardize the data for age and sex by applying appropriate weighting to age/sex bands in the practice. The method for doing this is not difficult, and is described in Kirkwood (1988).

Interpreting changes in physiological measurements

It is quite usual to select a group of patients with high values of a particular measurement—for example blood pressure or cholesterol—and then follow them up later to see whether their readings have improved. Interpreting the results of this exercise presents a particular difficulty because of a phenomenon known as 'regression to the mean'. Because of the natural variation in an individual's blood pressure or cholesterol reading, whenever a group of patients with high values are followed up, their repeat results will, on average, always be lower than before. This means that if patients with high blood pressure or high cholesterol are identified and followed up later they inevitably appear to be doing well, even though there may have been no effective intervention at all (see example p. 234). The extent of this 'regression to the mean' can be greater than any anticipated clinical effect. Note than regression to the mean also works in the opposite direction, so that a group of patients with unusually low readings to start with will always have higher readings, on average, at follow-up.

Repeated measurements of blood pressure may be affected by yet another phenomenon—that of accommodation. An individual's blood pressure will tend to reduce on repeated readings as he or she gets more used to the procedure. This means that the average blood pressure of any group on remeasurement may be about 4.0/2.0 mmHg lower than at the first reading (Rose *et al.* 1980).

The extent of accommodation and regression to the mean was demonstrated by recruitment to the Medical Research Council Trial of mild hypertension (MRC Working Party 1985). Patients were only admitted to the trial if both the mean of three readings by a nurse and of two further readings by a doctor were within the required range. Yet at each annual follow-up for five years, 40 per cent of those on placebo had diastolic blood pressure below the admission level of 90 mmHg.

CONCLUSIONS

Collecting and interpreting data for audit can be stimulating and enjoyable if you choose an interesting and important question and carry out the audit with reasonable care. Data collection which is not well planned is depressing because it takes time and then produces a result which is not relevant or precise enough to form a basis for change and planning for future care. The simple skills described in this chapter are far from exhaustive, but are intended to give some idea of what is meant by 'reasonable care' and 'well planned' and also to encourage further reading.

In the end, audit skills will be learnt by practical experience rather than by reading books. But there are general questions which could reasonably be asked of most audits to assess 'reasonable care'.

1. Are rates reported?
2. Are the denominators clinically sensible?
3. Is ascertainment of the denominators complete?
4. Is the sample adequate to provide confidence in the result?

In addition, when making comparisons over time, three further questions must be asked:

1. Is the change firmly attributable to the effect of medical care?
2. Has the effect of random variation been considered?
3. Has regression to the mean been excluded as a cause for change?

Members of primary health care teams who conduct audits and can say that they have considered and dealt with these questions will achieve a believable result on which changes in clinical practice can safely be initiated.

REFERENCES

Coulter, A. Rowland, M., and Wilkin, D. (1991). *GP referrals to hospital—a guide for Family Health Service Authorities*. Centre for Primary Care Research, Manchester.
Coulter, A., Bradlow, J., Martin-Bates, C., Agass, M., and Tulloch, A. (1992). Outcome of general practitioner referrals to specialist outpatient clinics for back pain. *British Journal of General Practice*, **41**, 450–3.
Gray, J. A. M., O'Dwyer, A., Fullard, E. M., and Fowler, G. H. (1987). Rent-an-audit. *Journal of the Royal College of General Practitioners*, **37**, 177.
Mant, D. and Tulloch, A. (1987). Completeness of chronic disease registration in general practice. *British Medical Journal*, **294**, 223–4.
Medical Research Council Working Party. (1985). MRC trial of mild hypertension: principal results. *British Medical Journal*, **291**, 97–104.
Rose, G., Heller, R. F., Tunstall Pedoe, H., and Christie, D. G. S. (1980). Heart disease prevention project: a randomised controlled trial in industry. *British Medical Journal*, **i**, 747–51.

FURTHER READING

General methodology

Armstrong, D., Calman, M., and Grace, J. (1990). *Research methods for general practitioners*. Oxford University Press.

General statistics

Kirkwood, B. (1988). *Essentials of medical statistics*. Blackwell, Oxford.

Natural variation

Theory

Ingelfinger, J., Mosteller, F., Thibodeau, L., and Ware, J. (1987). *Biostatistics in clinical medicine*. MacMillan, New York.

Interpretation of referral rates

Roland, M. O., Bartholomew, J., Morrell, D. C. *et al.* (1990). Understanding hospital referral rates: a user's guide. *British Medical Journal*, **301**, 98–102.

Sampling

Kahn, H. and Sempos, C. (1989). *Statistical methods in epidemiology*. (Chapter 2), Oxford University Press, New York.

Questionnaire design

Theory

Moser, C. and Kalton, G. (1978). *Survey methods in social investigation*. Heinemann, Oxford.

Inspiration

Cartwright, A. (1988). *Health surveys in practice and potential*. King's Fund, London.
Wilkin, D., Hallam, L., and Doggett, M. (1992). *Measures of need and outcome in primary health care*. Oxford University Press.

Measurement

Honey, S. and Cummings, R. (ed.) (1988). *Design in clinical research* (Chapters 4 and 5) Williams and Wilkins, Baltimore.

APPENDIX

Sample size

The sample size required is calculated from the formula:

$$n = \frac{1.96^2 \, N \, p \, (1 - p)}{1.96^2 \, p \, (1 - p) + \Delta^2 \, N}$$

Where Δ = range of accuracy required:

(0.025 for ± 2.5 per cent; 0.05 for ± 5.0 per cent)

p = a priori estimate of the proportion meeting the audit criterion.

N = number of patients to be audited.

1.96 is the constant for 95 per cent confidence. (This is the usually recommended level. It can be replaced by 1.645 for 90 per cent confidence).

Error attached to sample results

If the sample proportion is p, the range of values within which, with 95 per cent probability, the population percentage will fall is:

$$p \pm 1.96 \sqrt{\frac{(p) \, (1 - p) \, (N - n)}{nN}}$$

When one sample result has an error of δ_1 and the other an error of δ_2, the error attached to the difference between sample results is $\sqrt{(\delta_1^2 + \delta_2^2)}$.

7 Implementing change and planning care

Peter Havelock

The process of bringing about change is based on simple, common sense theory, but the implementation of that theory is complex and riddled with hazards. It involves a move from collecting, collating, and presenting data to an alteration of behaviour in the practice to improve the quality of care (Rogers 1971).

In the introduction to Part II the characteristics of a healthy practice were outlined. Those characteristics allow a practice to perform effectively and the time and effort expended in attaining them are well rewarded. Often such ideal circumstances are unobtainable; for instance, due to a long history of resistance to change within the practice, or due to one powerful partner blocking all progress. If these or other similar circumstances apply to you, do not be put off introducing audit. Often the process of examining the quality of the care you provide, including team work, discussion, planning, and effective meetings can help to bring about the metamorphosis to a healthier practice. If you are the person trying to introduce change into your practice do not get too disheartened by initial resistance and failures, but use the ideas and principles in the following chapter to help 'sell' your ideas to the other members of your practice.

BRINGING ABOUT CHANGE

Change is about making a journey from the position where you are now to a redefined position sometime in the future. As in making a journey, all the people who are going on the trip need to be involved at each stage. The route needs to be planned and changed if necessary. Hazards need to be identified, and plans for overcoming them made. Recalcitrant members may need help and support. A leader is needed, with the vision of where everyone is going. Other people help and may modify the route—for example, the navigators, the pilot, look-outs to watch for hazards and show people the path. There needs to be a back marker to make sure that nobody is left behind, and that people are not going in the wrong direction. Somebody must look after the welfare of the travellers, because moving and travelling can be stressful.

The analogy of the journey is applicable to all organizations, but is especially apt in the smaller service ones, such as general practice.

EFFECTIVE LEADERSHIP

The successful introduction of audit into practice needs leadership, sometimes by a group of people, but more often by one person. Much has been written about effective leadership, but probably the clearest and most useful account is in *Leading in the NHS—a practical guide* by Rosemary Stewart (1989). She states that an effective leader should:

(1) point the way—a good leader provides the vision;
(2) symbolize what matters—a leader embodies the values and the meaning of the practice, and shows clearly what he or she cares about;
(3) get others to share the ideals—sharing vision is so very important in effecting change;
(4) create pride in the organization—the members of a practice will achieve higher standards if they know what they do well and are proud of it;
(5) make people feel important—the practice members will have more energy and will set themselves higher standards if they know that they, and what they do, matter.
(6) realize people's potential—all human beings have a great deal of unrealized potential; the effective leader enables the practice members to release that energy;
(7) self-sufficiency—being a leader can be lonely; it is this that makes many withdraw from leadership.

Stewart (1989) concludes 'Many readers could lead provided they know what they want to achieve and could communicate it to others.'

SHARING INFORMATION

The choice of subject has been made, the current performance has been observed, and on the basis of this information, necessary changes need to be agreed and future care planned. The data can be presented to the practice in a number of different ways, some may be more acceptable to members of the practice than others. Presentation of raw data can produce resistance, because the recipients may not understand, may misinterpret, or fail to appreciate the implications of the findings. Probably the most effective method of stimulating planning and change is to present the objective figures simply and clearly, and offer comments and conclusions that are recognized as both personal and subjective.

For example, the results of an audit of unwanted pregnancies that shows patchy family planning delivery might be presented to the practice, with suggestions of using a record card together with some examples and perhaps an article about the number and effect of unplanned pregnancies. The figures, the comments, and the conclusions are then available for the practice to discuss.

From this discussion the general direction of change can be determined. In order to have any success, all those who are affected by the audit and its implications will need to be involved from the start; for example, it would be difficult to audit accessibility without involving the receptionists and all the doctors at all stages.

The process of change can be summarized as follows:

Strategy $\rightarrow$ Plan $\rightarrow$ Implementation $\rightarrow$ Changed behaviour and commitment

(Preparation)   (The journey)   (The destination)

PLANNING IN GENERAL PRACTICE

With the constant pressures of patient demand and the preoccupation with the day to day running of the practice, it is not surprising that so few general practices have either the mechanism or the time to plan for developments that are more than a few months ahead. Planning needs to be seen in two ways.

1. Strategic planning—a long-term look at where the practice is going, and how it might get there. The time scale is longer than that which is going to be done in next week or next month, but if longer than 2—3 years it is unlikely to be realistic, it enters the realm of 'crystal ball gazing'.
2. Tactical planning—the day to day planning that is necessary to run the practice. This is the usual activity of most practice meetings. The time scale is often very short, with a definite purpose in mind.

A number of activities can aid a practice in planning. They are described briefly here, but greater detail can be found in a variety of management books (see further reading list).

Agreeing a purpose

Any practice reviewing the management of a topic of care must decide what they are trying to achieve in handling that topic—otherwise it is impossible to decide how to achieve it.

Visioning

The practice members should share their visions of good care, even if they are not immediately attainable, so that they can develop a common aim and plan for the future.

Brainstorming

The group gathers all ideas about a subject that can be recorded, often on a flip chart, without comment or criticism, until all the ideas are collected. They can then be grouped and discussed. This enables everyone to enter into the decision making process.

Force field analysis

Once you know where you want to go, this helps to plan the way to get there. The group identifies those forces that are helping change, and those forces that are resisting. Discussion within the partnership, identifying the resisting forces, and helping to reduce or redirect them, can be very fruitful.

SWOT analysis

This is another technique for exploring the potential for and obstacles to change within the practice. It is the analysis of the aspects of change in relationship to the practice and its members.

> Strengths
> Weaknesses
> Opportunities — for whom?
> Threats   — to whom?

The likely effect of the change on members of the practice can be predicted, problems forecasted, and sorted out.

To bring about change, both strategic and tactical planning are necessary, but most important is the strategic planning, which general practitioners often find so difficult. To return to the analogy of the journey, it is useful and helpful to have all the crew members involved at the beginning, but it is essential that all the officers agree about the major parts of the plan, especially the desired destination. In general practice, the partners need to have a vision of where they are going and plan for getting there. Sharing this vision and plan requires a commitment of time and effective communication between all the team members. The essential starting point is the practice meeting.

EFFECTIVE PRACTICE MEETINGS

There are a wide variety of meetings that come under the general heading of 'practice meetings', ranging through a brief chat over coffee, a partner's meeting, a meeting of a subgroup dealing with a particular topic, or a team meeting including all of the attached staff. These meetings serve different functions and as such all are important.

The reason for the meeting

There is no value in meeting for meeting's sake. Each meeting must have objectives, and these will determine the nature of the meeting. Choosing the type of sterilizer or the colour of the curtains can often be done at routine meetings, often with long agendas, or on some occasions be delegated to others. More important subjects, such as setting up a diabetic clinic, or changing the appointment system, require more time, perhaps a meeting dedicated to one topic. The right people need to attend, preparation must be careful, and effective chairing and recording of the meeting is esential in obtaining and agreeing good decisions.

Timing the meeting

Pressures of patients and time can often displace the meetings till late at night after a busy day, or in a lunchtime, with partners arriving late or leaving early. When planning the future of the practice, time needs to be set aside so that everyone is able to concentrate fully on the issues involved. Some practices now regularly allocate a day or half a day away from the workplace, with a locum looking after the patients, so that the partners have the freedom to plan effectively.

The agenda

This is the written timetable for the meeting, covering all the subjects that are to be discussed. The agenda, together with a paper of explanation including the audit results and suggested points for discussion, ensures participants are informed, and important decisions can be made more effectively. The agenda and audit results should be sent out long enough before the meeting, so that all those attending can gather their thoughts and thus join in the discussion.

Role of chairperson

A good chairperson structures discussion, allows a free flow of relevant ideas, assists the groups towards making a decision, interprets, clarifies, moves the discussion forward, and brings it to a resolution which everybody understands and accepts as the general consensus of the meeting, even if not everyone is necessarily in full agreement. The chairperson is not there to impose his or her will on the meeting or limit the free flow of ideas, indeed it is probably better if the major advocate or protagonist of an idea is not the chairperson of that meeting. In partnerships, the chairperson is often the senior partner, which may make the problem of control and equitable discussion difficult. Discussion within the partnership about the role of chairperson, and the best person to manage that role most effectively, can be very fruitful.

Recording the meeting

The minutes of the meeting should record the decisions made, the person responsible for carrying them out, and by what time and date. They can then be consulted subsequently when promoting action within the practice. The minutes should be written and shared with all people concerned.

THE CARE PLAN

Once agreed, the plans need to be clear and written down in the form of guidelines.

The ingredients of a care plan

1. Definition of topic or target group of patients.
2. Aims of care.
3. Roles of team members.
4. Structure
    (a) equipment
    (b) records
    (c) accessibility
    (d) patient information
    (e) training.
5. Process or procedures of care.
6. Targets or outcomes.
7. Criteria and method of review.
8. Timetable for implementation and review.

These ingredients are required to plan both clinical care, for example a diabetic clinic, or to implement changes in practice organization, for example the appointment system.

IMPLEMENTATION OF THE CARE PLAN—MANAGEMENT OF CHANGE

Perhaps the most difficult part of the whole audit cycle is turning the plan into action, that is making the journey from where you are now to where you want to be into the future. A number of components need to be considered if the implementation of planning and change is to be effective:

(1) clarity of plans;
(2) a shared vision of the future;
(3) operating principles;
(4) environment of change;
(5) transition management;
(6) resistance reduction;
(7) commitment planning.

Clarity of plans

Often we make plans which we understand fully when we make them, but which appear confused and muddled on transmission to the other members of the practice team. There is no substitute for written plans that everyone can read and comment on. If they are not clear, the plans need changing. A confusing map is often worse than no map at all.

For example, a plan for recruiting patients to a well-person clinic will clearly state the role of each team member and the actions that each should perform.

A shared vision of the future

If all the practice members have a similar view about what they want the practice to achieve then they are more likely to agree on a plan that moves them towards that vision. The key is the involvement of all the members of the practice in planning and change. Involvement means much more than telling other people what to do, it means sharing ideas and getting feedback on those ideas from everyone. Involvement takes time, effort, and skill but it is essential if commitment to change is to be achieved.

For example, everyone in the team will wish to improve the quality of service and accessibility of the practice to patients, and so members of the team should feel competent to deal with their particular responsibility in running the appointment system and answering the telephone.

Operating principles

The practice's working principles guide the members through complex and conflicting choices: examples could include:

1. We wish to provide the highest quality of care for patients
2. We wish that all members of staff enjoy their job.
3. We wish to maximize the income of the partners.
4. Routine surgery work should be completed before 6.30 pm.

Operating principles can conflict with each other and these conflicts need to be resolved by the partners. It helps other practice members if the principles are made explicit and thus some decisions can be made by the staff more easily.

For example, operating principles in the care of diabetes can vary: from 'We believe that diabetes is a disease to be looked after by specialists in hospital', to 'We believe that diabetes is a disease of primary care with the hospital only being involved for severe complications'. Or from 'We believe that suitably trained nurses are able to care for most problems of diabetic patients', to 'We believe that doctors are the most appropriate people to look after diabetic patients'. The awareness and understanding of operating principles demonstrated in this example must be applied throughout all the practice work.

Environment of change

The environment of practice can be subdivided into the external and internal environment.

The external environment, following the introduction of the new contract, has put both pressures and opportunities on to practices. The pressures are easy to identify: more data recording, meeting targets, routine three-yearly checks and elderly surveillance. Examples of opportunities might be: fewer restrictions on types of staff, enabling the employment of a practice counsellor; opportunities for staff education; PACT information more freely available, enabling the practice to develop a formulary.

The internal environment of the practice includes the sorts of things that make the practice healthy or unhealthy (pp. 33–6). A key test of the internal environment of the practice is the extent to which the practice has responded to change in the past.

If, for example, the internal environment of the practice is such that the partners do not share the care of chronically sick patients with the nurse or even with each other, it will be more difficult to bring about a co-ordinated programme of care for any group of patients, for example, hypertensive patients, diabetic patients, or women on hormone replacement therapy.

Transition management

Any journey needs managing. If allowed to happen in a haphazard manner a number of things can occur. Some people arrive in the wrong place, some give up and go home, some go on, some fall by the wayside. Bringing about change needs active management and work; in management terms the journey is described as a transition state.

In general practice the development and acceptance of the care plan and then its implementation by modification of clinical practice is the transition state. Practice members need help moving through these stages to see the benefits of the new way of working. They may need extra time and resources to allow the new working practices to be adopted—time for meetings and discussion, resources for new equipment. Often the plan can be guided through by the practice subgroup that has been particularly responsible for the topic, a subgroup which involves representatives of those most involved in the change.

For example, in setting up a family planning clinic; the team might consist of a doctor, practice nurse, and practice manager. In reviewing the availability of appointments; the appropiate team might be a receptionist, doctor, and the practice manager.

Successful management of transition needs to involve all practice members, but in particular those member whose opinions are well respected within the practice—the opinion leaders. To get these opinion leaders on board at an early stage will smooth the passage of the change considerably.

Reducing the resistance to change

Although there are usually obvious benefits to be gained by change, people may also experience a sense of loss in the process. The fear of this loss and the perception of the loss can engender resistance. The loss can be of different types:

1. Security or control—any change in a work pattern is a step into the unknown. Staff may be concerned that it will involve more work, they will not have adequate time, there may not be financial recognition, they may even become redundant.
2. Competence—people might need new skills, which as yet they do not have and which makes them feel less than competent to do the new job.
3. Relationships—the change might mean the loss of previous arrangements, relationships, or working patterns.
4. Sense of direction—because the situation around them is changing, people might not know where they are going or what might happen next.
5. Territory—the change might bring about alterations in the use of space and people might lose their familiar patch.

These losses or potential losses need to be recognized and acknowledged by the practice and if possible kept to a minimum. When asked to change people tend to go through four phases.

1. Denial—this is initial numbness, particularly over major changes. People go on working as if nothing is going to change. Communication and discussion at an early stage with the involvement of the whole practice in the decision making can minimize this phase.
2. Resistance—this can occur when people have moved through the numbness of denial and begin to experience self doubt, anger, depression, anxiety, frustration, fear, or uncertainty because of the changes. Again, early involvement and discussion helps people through this. It helps if the change can be reduced to a series of small steps, so that people can comprehend and achieve each stage as they make the transition. Each step can be worked through with the people involved and adapted to suit them if appropriate.

For example, as a result of an audit the practice may wish to improve the quality of its asthma care. Instead of rushing in to set up a nurse run asthma clinic, the practice might introduce a record card first, then regular review, then a joint doctor/nurse clinic, and, finally, a nurse run asthma clinic. This will allow doctors, nurses, reception staff, and patients time to get used to the change and to gather expertise as necessary.

In their book *Management in general practice* Pritchard *et al.* (1984) wrote 'People may resist change because:

(a) they are anxious or threatened — discuss and reassure
(b) they are apathetic — may need encouragement
(c) they are confused — discuss and clarify
(d) there is nothing in it for them — replan so that there is.'

3. Exploration — at this point people are becoming positive to the change and looking towards the future. It is important to capitalize on this energy and enthusiasm and give those members of staff with good ideas and enthusiasm the freedom to develop and grow with the change. Inspired leadership is required to channel and encourage the practice in the new development.
4. Commitment — this is the final stage. Change is fully introduced and part of the standard operating procedure of the practice.

Planning for commitment

The final stage of change within practice is the commitment of everybody to the inclusion of the new methods into their work. This is the end point of the journey, the destination, and unless people arrive there, all the planning and implementation is lost. It is important to remember that unless behaviour changes nothing changes.

Many times in practice a new idea is introduced, people agree to it and maybe start, but then they revert back to the previous patterns of behaviour. Certain activities can increase commitment to change.

1. Early identification and solving of problems.
2. A reward system that recognizes the new working conditions. For example, extra hours set aside for an asthma clinic and maybe an increase in grade for the practice nurse in view of the new work.
3. Educational activity. Appropriate education can help people overcome the lack of competence that they feel as a result of the new working conditions.
4. Role modelling. If the doctors do not adopt the new procedures it is unlikely that other members of the practice will either. It is not a coincidence that polite, considerate doctors have friendly, courteous receptionists.

To get a practice committed to, for example, a new diabetic policy and protocol everyone needs to be involved at every step; the doctors need to give up their 'clinical freedom' and agree a joint policy; the nurses need to feel confident in their role or acquire training to achieve it; and the receptionists need to be happy with the booking procedure. Commitment to the plan needs to be checked repeatedly with all groups during the transition.

CONCLUSION

Change is happening in practice all the time. At this time of the new general practice contract, the external pressures of change are greater than they have been for years. Audit will produce further pressures of change, an internal pressure, a pressure to improve the quality of care within the practice.

The change needs to be planned, the transition state needs to be managed and new operating procedures in the practice need to be adopted. Such developments require an open, involving type of leadership, and the doctors themselves need a cohesive shared vision of the future. All such skills take time to acquire, but time and effort at an early stage will earn rewards in many changes to come.

REFERENCES AND FURTHER READING

Plant, R. (1987). *Managing change and making it stick*. Fontana/Collins, London.
Pritchard, P., Low, K., and Whalen, M. (1984). *Management in general practice*. Oxford University Press.
Rogers, E. M. (1987). *Diffusion of innovations*. Free Press Collier MacMillan, London.
Stewart, R. (1989). Leading in the NHS, a practical guide. MacMillan, London.
Turril, A. (1986). *Change and innovation, a challenge for the NHS*. Management Series 10, Institute of Health Service Management, London.

8 Repeating the cycle

Martin Lawrence

It is widely agreed that the most important aspect of audit is the production of change and improvement in patient services. Assessment of such change, and guarantee of its persistence, can only be ensured by regular review of activity. The question becomes not so much *why* one should do repeated audit, but rather *how* it can be included in a crowded practice schedule. After a brief review of the reasons for recommending a cyclical approach for audit, this chapter will concentrate mainly on how it can be achieved.

WHY REPEAT THE CYCLE?

Accountability

With primary care teams increasingly being accountable to patients for services and to government for use of resources it is essential that the service is regularly reviewed, and seen to be reviewed. It is neither necessary nor possible to audit every aspect of care, but enough tracer conditions need to be covered to provide assurance that the whole practice is likely to be of comparable standard.

Implement change

The most common failing in audit is that practices collect data but do not act on them. A subject is chosen, data collected, discussed (often only by the doctors), and filed. The same subject may be examined again later in the same way, but such data collection may not imply repeating the cycle, there may just be a short circuit of part of the cycle, as illustrated in Fig. 8.1.

To ensure change and improvement, it is necessary for each stage of the cycle to be passed through. Evaluation must be followed by consideration of change, the drawing up of a care plan, agreement on criteria for assessment, and *then* returning to data collection. An audit which does not produce or change a plan for care is of little value.

Setting targets

The entry point into the cycle is of no importance only if the cycle is completed. Whereas assessment theoretically begins with the development of criteria, the cycle can be entered anywhere, in the sure knowledge that this will take place

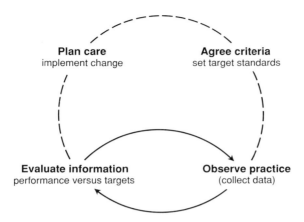

Fig. 8.1 A short-cut in the audit cycle.

eventually so long as the cycle is adhered to. Without target standards the care will remain undirected and evaluation will be impossible. One is reminded of the aphorism about Christopher Columbus 'When he set out he didn't know where he was going, when he got there he didn't know where he was, and when he came home he didn't know where he'd been'.

Very few practices know what targets they can, or even should achieve. Guidance in setting targets for the practice can be derived from the literature, or by reference to evidence of local performance or agreement, but for each individual practice realistic targets have to be assessed in the light of current achievement. Repeating the cycle gives the opportunity of refining the criteria and changing the target levels of performance. Target standards should be developed and then reviewed after each cycle of audit.

Longitudinal care

General practice is carried out on a longitudinal, rather than a cross-sectional basis. Individual patient care may go on over years. This gives a unique opportunity not only to maintain and improve services generally, but even to review the care of individuals on a repeated basis (see 'heart sink' patients, p. 153).

Morale

Members of primary health care teams work very hard, often it seems for poor return. This is especially because benefits due to therapy in primary care are often small; and many of the results are in things that do not happen—the strokes that do not happen because of blood pressure treatment, or the abortions that do not happen because of good family planning. To help staff and doctors see the benefit of their work it is necessary to provide formal evaluation.

Quality assurance

In the best of systems standards can slip, improvements slide away. The only way to ensure that we maintain the highest quality is to continue to examine it.

HOW CAN REPEATING THE CYCLE BE MADE EASIER?

Setting priorities

Taking on new audits, but at the same time repeating all previous ones appears to imply a relentless increase in the workload. We need to look for ways in which such workload can be moderated.

It is important to agree *how often* the audit of a topic needs to be repeated. This will depend on how important an item of care it is, and how adequate was the care revealed by the previous audit. The practice may agree that an important topic in which many care changes have been made may need reviewing in six months or a year; whereas a smaller problem where the care is good, or where changes have been made resulting in good care as evidenced by one repeat audit, may not need to be revisited for several years.

For example, one can contrast the diabetic audit (pp. 128–9), where a practice has been struggling to improve care in a major area and only gradually obtaining improvement, so needing regular review; with the warfarin audit (pp. 161–2), where a practice with a problem made a few specific changes and on review found the care to be foolproof.

It may also be that a less extensive audit can sometimes be carried out. If a major review had involved data collection, a practice meeting, care plan agreement, and setting of target standards, then some time later a sub-team might just look at data, confirm that the targets are being met, and leave detailed evaluation on that occasion.

Involving the whole team

It is becoming increasingly common for a records officer to be employed for the express purpose of conducting audits; or the practice manager or a member of staff can have time dedicated to audit. That person becomes well versed in audit methodology, adept at manipulating records and computer data, skilled in interpreting data, and so able to take responsibility for implementing regular audit.

Whether or not the primary health care team includes a records officer, regular audit can be helped by spreading the work around the practice. This has several benefits:

1. Everyone does some work, but nobody does too much.
2. There is a learning opportunity for all team members, and each member has the chance to use different skills.
3. If data collection and analysis is undertaken by staff then the partners are less reluctant to undertake new audits, and can devote their energy and skills to planning change and setting target standards.
4. Morale is raised by enabling team members to become more involved in the performance of the practice.
5. There is greater potential for improving the service, because more members of the team are looking at each topic, each from their own perspective.

In the author's practice this has been done, with a member of staff responsible for each topic which is regularly audited, while a partner provides resource and support. In addition, the time of the year when each data collection should be completed is stipulated, so spreading the work through the year (Table 8.1). An example is the diabetic audit on pp. 128–9, which in 1991 was conducted and presented to the practice meeting entirely by a receptionist.

While this arrangement covers the regular audit of important topics, it also spreads the workload so that team members still have time and energy occasionally to undertake a 'critical event audit'.

Improving records

The more organized are the records, the quicker it is to search the notes—it is certainly much easier to check data on a flow card than by working through all the continuation sheets.

Table 8.1 *An example schedule for data collection and analysis*

Topic	Staff member	Doctor	Date
Child care/immunization	Health visitor	A	May
Hypertension clinic	Nurse X	B	October
Diabetic care	Receptionist G	B	January
Access	Receptionist H	B	March and September
Continuity of care	Receptionist H	B	December and June
Registration	Receptionist J	A	January
Health checks	Nurse Y	C	October
New patient checks	Nurse Y	C	November
More than 75 checks	Nurse Z	C	April
Well-women clinic	Nurse X	D	April
Cervical smears	Receptionist J	D	Quarterly
Pharmacy/formulary	Receptionist K	A	April
Practice report	Practice Manager	C	March/April

Data can be collected *regularly and routinely* with audit in mind. Work load figures can be collected daily by reception staff: cardiac risk factors can be entered on a pro forma at each health promotion clinic so that change can be monitored without the need to retrieve notes.

In many computerized practices data can be entered directly during consultation and is then available for analysis, but to make the exercise successful the practice must agree on uniform behaviour. Preventive and chronic disease management procedures must be entered on every occasion: diagnostic criteria must be uniform so that disease registers can be produced: and referral or visit data will be meaningless if they are not complete.

Repeating an audit can be helped by filing the protocol and data collection forms after each cycle. this both saves a great deal of time and effort when the audit is next performed, and also ensures that the data is collected in the same way each time. Computerized practices have one special advantage—the computer can be programmed to repeat the same audit at regular intervals, perhaps even overnight. Three examples can be cited.

1. Many computers can be used with report generator software. The practice can design computer searches and store them in the report generator, which then carries out the search in an identical manner at pre-programmed intervals. This offers great flexibility for individual practices.
2. Practices can combine to use the same audit programme. For example, the Wycombe computing project involves 21 practices using Update computers (Trower 1990). One member of the group designs audit searches which are reviewed and agreed by the group. Once adopted, the same audit programme is installed in each practice, so not only is data collected regularly but practices can compare results.
3. An audit programme can be developed by a computer firm on the advice of its user group and inserted to the software of all user practices who can then run it if they wish. Such an exercise has been carried out by the author in conjunction with VAMP, and the result of this audit in 38 practices caring for 430 000 patients has been reported (Lawrence *et al.* 1990). This system offers no flexibility to individuals, but has great potential for stimulating discussion by comparing performance between practices.

EVALUATION AND PLANNING

We have taken care throughout this book to emphasize that data collection is not audit, it is only one component. Yet it is often the most time consuming element, the stage which holds practices up for fear of the workload. For this reason this chapter has concentrated on the collection of data.

For effective audit, which involves producing change and setting targets, it is essential that practice procedures are set up to consider the data and act on it.

A great deal of that process has been considered in Chapter 4, but it is worth emphasizing a few points necessary to ensure effective audit activities persist.

1. An individual or group in the practice must be responsible for the collation and presentation of the data. Increasingly this will be a records officer. Certainly the person may not be a doctor, but if an individual is not responsible then the activity will very likely lapse.
2. It may be helpful for that individual to have the support of a small team who take an interest in that particular topic. They can examine the data in detail and develop proposals to put to the practice; and they can be responsible for implementing any decisions for change taken by the practice.
3. A formal session will be made necessary for the data to be presented to the whole practice team. This could occur as one of a regular series of practice education meetings. In this way everyone sees the results of their work and can offer opinions on present achievements, and suggestions for improvement. Such meetings maximize the opportunity of getting everyone working together for improvement, and they improve morale and motivation due to a feeling of 'ownership'.
4. After practice discussion, it will probably be more appropriate for the small group formally to draw up any new plans for care and target standards — the whole practice can be unwieldly for such an activity. And so the cycle begins again.

Remember: an audit which does not produce a plan is of little value, and target standards should be developed and reviewed after each cycle of audit.

REFERENCES

Trower, C. (1990). Organising for quality: Wycombe Primary Care Computing. *Practice Computing*, September, 13–15.

Lawrence, M. S., Coulter, A., and Jones, L. (1990). A total audit of preventive procedures in 45 practices caring for 430,000 patients. *British Medical Journal*, **300**, 510–13.

Part III
Audit in practice

9 Preventive care: child surveillance and women's health

Mary Pierce

CHILD HEALTH SURVEILLANCE AND IMMUNIZATION

Choosing the topic

The foundations of our current child health services lie in the dreadful mortality figures of the end of the last century. In 1900 in Nottingham 161 per 1000 children died within their first year of life. By 1922 a child welfare service had been started. In 1967 the Sheldon Report recommended a series of checks which have been repeated almost continuously since then (Sheldon Report 1967).

The Royal College of General Practitioners report *Healthier children — thinking prevention* strongly advocated the early integration of developmental surveillance into general practice (Royal College of General Practitioners 1982). In 1989 a review of child health surveillance *Health for all children* (Hall 1990, 2nd edn) critically appraised current activities and made recommendations as to whether practices should be continued or discontinued.

The contract for general practice (Department of Health and the Welsh Office 1989) introduced in 1990 has furthered these initiatives and encourages general practitioners to take over child health surveillance, as an integral part of primary care. These developments mean that it is a most opportune time for general practitioners to be auditing child surveillance services. The case for auditing immunization rates is even stronger. It is unarguably a service producing direct benefits to patients, and since the 1990 contract the practice will receive a payment if 70 per cent or 90 per cent of the necessary vaccinations have been administered to 2-year-old children.

Developing a practice policy for care

Practice policies for these activities must be agreed, preferably at a meeting for all those involved in child health surveillance and immunization. A good start is to debate an existing set of guidelines: this might be obtained from your local FHSA, District Health Authority, or from the *The child surveillance handbook* (Hall *et al.* 1990), or by using Table 9.1.

Agreeing vaccination policy is less problematic as there are clear national guidelines (Table 9.2).

Developing target standards

Target standards, i.e. criteria used for assessment and levels of performance, should cover any areas where the team feel there are problems in the service, and should be relevant and important. They should be developed for the practice, though the team may well decide to adopt or adapt criteria already used elsewhere.

Such criteria for assessment of immunization are relatively unambiguous — they relate to ensuring that the immunization has been given (Table 9.3).

Table 9.1 *Recommended procedures for child health surveillance (after Hall et al. 1990)*

Age	Procedure
6 weeks	Check history and ask about parental concerns.
	Physical examination, weight, head circumference.
	Check for congenital dislocation of hip.
	Inspect the eyes.
	Ask about parental concerns on vision and hearing.
	Advise parents about detection of hearing loss.
8 months (range 7–9 months)	Ask about parental concerns, particularly regarding vision and hearing.
	Check weight if indicated.
	Check for evidence of congenital dislocation of hip.
	Check for testicular descent in boys.
	Observe visual behaviour and examine for squint.
	Carry out distraction test for hearing.
21 months (range 18–24 months)	Ask about parental concerns, particularly regarding vision and hearing.
	Confirm that the child is:
	walking normally
	beginning to say words
	understands when spoken to.
	Remember high prevalence of iron-deficiency anaemia.
39 months (range 36–42 months)	Check vision, squint, hearing, behaviour, and development, and refer as appropriate.
	Measure height and plot on chart.
	Check for testicular descent.
	Check immunization status.

For child health surveillance the problem is more complex (Table 9.4). The practice may start by reviewing the process of care by ensuring that children are seen and examined. Once these criteria have been achieved the practice may wish to proceed to outcome criteria (Table 9.5). Criteria may get more rigorous as the practice achieves the simpler ones.

Once criteria are agreed, the practice team must decide what level of performance is ideal or desired. What is achievable in a population for the same amount of effort is very different in a middle class affluent area from a deprived inner city area, but that is not to say that ideal standards cannot be met in a deprived population with more effort and some lateral thinking. Nevertheless a

Table 9.2 *Recommended immunization schedule for children under 5 years old (UK 1990)*

Age	Immunization
2 months	1st diphtheria, tetanus, pertussis and polio (DTPPol)
3 months	2nd DTPPol
4 months	3rd DTPPol
13 months	measles, mumps and rubella (MMR)
4½ years	Booster DTPPol

Table 9.3 *Suggested criteria for auditing immunization in children under 5 years of age*

1. All 2-year-olds should have had three doses of vaccine for diphtheria, tetanus, and polio, unless medically contraindicated.
2. All 2-year-olds should have had three doses of pertussis vaccine.
3. All 2-year-olds should have had one dose of MMR vaccine.
4. All 5-year-olds should have had a pre-school booster of diphtheria, tetanus, and polio vaccine.

Table 9.4 *Suggestions for criteria of process which might be used for an audit of child health surveillance*

1. A child reaching one year of age should have had the newborn, 6 weeks, and 8 months checks.
2. A 2-year-old child should have had its 18 month check.
3. A 4-year-old child should have had its 3 years and over check.
4. A child attending any given clinic should have the agreed procedures carried out.

Table 9.5 *Outcome criteria which might be used for audit of child health surveillance*

---

1. A child's parents should know the importance of checking for deafness and how to do it.
2. A child should not have congenital dislocation of the hip (CDH) diagnosed after the age of 6 months.
3. A child should not reach the age of 4½ years with undiagnosed squint or amblyopia.
4. Any child found to have a hearing difficulty should have been fully evaluated and followed up.

---

practice may legitimately feel that an ideal level of performance is unachievable at present, in which case the practice should set its target level between the current and the ideal. In this way the team may be encouraged by demonstrable improvement in their quality of care, and targets which earlier may have seemed unattainable may be achieved.

Collecting and analysing the data

Collecting data for immunization and child health surveillance is usually straightforward, because such data should be recorded routinely in each patient's notes. This will have required some double entry with health visitor and/or patient carried notes, but unless it is done, the practice will have no record for clinical care or audit and should re-examine its procedures.

Tabulation of results on a regular basis can be done *either* by computer search *or* by extracting the notes of the relevant age band of children. This may well be done by involving the health visitor for the practice.

In this way the practice may produce a table giving the percentage of:

1. Children age 2 years, fully immunized to DTPPol.
2. Children age 2 years, fully immunized to pertussis.
3. Children age 2 years, fully immunized to MMR.
4. Children age 5 years, fully immunized to DTPol.
5. Children age 1 year, up to date with child health surveillance and procedures carried out.
6. Children age 2 years, up to date with child health surveillance and procedures carried out.
7. Children age 4 years, up to date with child health surveillance and procedures carried out.

Observing the practice for outcomes may require a case discussion of significant rare events — for example, a child found amblyopic — or a note search on a sample to see whether clinical findings (such as hearing problems) are being dealt with and followed up.

Managing change

The findings will surely show that:

1. Certain children are behind with immunizations.
2. Certain children are not attending for child health surveillance.
3. Certain clinical procedures have been missed.
4. Certain clinical findings have not been followed up.

This exercise will give the practice a chance to catch up on those children who have been missed, but also to examine the management plan and the criteria for assessment. For instance:

1. Were they invited?

   The practice may need to modify the invitation system. One person should be responsible for inviting children at the appropriate ages. First and second postal invitations should, if necessary, be followed up by personal invitation from the health visitor. If these strategies fail to work the medical records should be tagged so that the issue can be raised by the doctor opportunistically the next time the child is seen in surgery. Finally, a home visit by the doctor may be necessary. (Parents do have a right to refuse to have their child subjected to child health surveillance and/or vaccination, so although a meticulous follow-up is recommended, it is not proposed that we oppress parents who have made up their minds not to have these procedures done.)

2. Are the times of the clinic convenient?

   Perhaps the practice needs to be more flexible about children visiting the clinic. Even a highly motivated parent can find it difficult to get a clinic appointment for the day when their child does not have a cold. After two or three attempts they inevitably become disheartened, especially if making these appointments involves taking time off work.

3. Were the children erroneously thought to have contraindications for vaccination, and/or are parents and medical workers inappropriately concerned about the safety of vaccines?

   In his analysis of the causes of failure of the British immunization campaign Nichol suggests professional ambiguity and ignorance as causes, and proposes a need for strong professional commitment to reach immunization targets (Nichol 1989). The practice may need to educate both the health care workers and parents. A continuous education campaign regarding vaccination may help. Antenatal classes are appropriate places to begin, and the Health Education Authority has excellent leaflets and posters to help.

4. Are the staff really committed to the protocols adopted?

If it is found that protocols agreed are not being completed this needs to be openly addressed and disagreements amicably settled. The Hall report's review of child health surveillance procedures and the new recommendations regarding timing of vaccinations have meant that procedures to which people had become attached over time had to be thrown out. This can cause resentment towards the new policies. Alternatively, are the protocols not being carried out because of lack of time or facilities? Or was it impossible to discover what had been done because of poor record keeping?

5. Should an opportunistic programme be blended into the clinic programme?

If notes of children who need child health surveillance or vaccination are tagged the doctor can use the opportunity of the next consultation in a regular surgery to doing the necessary examination or vaccination. This has been shown to be feasible and effective (Houston *et al.* 1990). Moreover, child health clinics may achieve greater attendance rates by offering therapeutic as well as preventive care (Rossdale *et al.* 1986).

Managing these sorts of changes can be difficult. No one person or group of people should be made to feel that not achieving targets is their fault. The team should be congratulated on its achievement so far and suggestions for improvement warmly welcomed.

The aim of the audit is to improve the quality of care and the group's enthusiasm and pride in its work. The whole practice team should become aware that vaccination and child health surveillance are not just things that the health visitors and clinic doctors do in well-baby clinics. It requires commitment from everyone in the practice. The receptionists should be helpful with information and 'fitting children in' to clinics. All health workers should be aware of the importance of accurate recording of information about child health surveillance and vaccination in the records and be constantly vigilant for children who have been missed.

Repeating the audit cycle

Having implemented these changes it is now necessary to repeat the examination of the notes or of the computer records to determine whether performance has improved. The whole audit cycle should be repeated as often as the group feels it is necessary.

Examples

Rossdale *et al.* described a well-baby clinic in a poor area of Britsol with very poor attendance and immunization rates. They identified serious problems and used many imaginative solutions to dramatic effect. The clinic was staffed with members of a primary health care team and a therapeutic service offered with a preventive service. Over a three year period they achieved an immunization rate of 95 per cent for diphtheria, tetanus, and polio and 93 per cent for measles. This is a heartening example to those struggling in the inner city (Rossdale *et al.* 1986).

A second example is of a study Curtis Jenkins did in his practice over a two year period. He concluded that child health surveillance was possible and feasible in general practice in co-operation with child health services. This is a good example of a descriptive audit and is full of ideas about improving attendance rates (Curtis Jenkins *et al.* 1978).

WOMENS' HEALTH: WELL-WOMEN'S CLINICS AND CERVICAL CYTOLOGY

Choosing the topic

It is particularly important to look at the quality of preventive services for women. More than half of a general practitioner's patients are female; women remain the custodians of families' health knowledge, so their attitudes to prevention will often determine their families' health care practices; women's lives tend to be highly medicalized—for much of their lives they are either taking contraception, pregnant, or menopausal, and when they are not consulting on their own behalf they are consulting about their children or other people for whom they care.

Prevention is fashionable, but the implicit assumption that preventive care is an unreserved good is being challenged. If a doctor is going to invite healthy patients to consult, offer advice about changing their life-styles, and expose them to screening procedures, then that doctor has responsibility for ensuring that only well-evaluated procedures of proven worth are carried out and that any pathology found is properly dealt with.

Some of what has been done in well-women's clinics has been found to be of little benefit, for example, breast self-examination (UK Trial of Early Detection of Breast Cancer 1988). Other procedures, for example cholesterol screening in women, have not been fully evaluated. However, Holland and Stewart (1990) provide a good critical analysis of the evidence for and against several screening procedures, and conclude that the evidence for both cervical cytology and mammography is strong.

Even well-evaluated procedures of proven worth will not work if an effective system is not developed to ensure that the appropriate people are reached. The

British National Cervical Cytology Scheme failed to produce a reduction in the mortality from carcinoma of the cervix in its first 20 years of operation. Many cervical smears were being done repeatedly on women at low risk.

Cervical cancer is an excellent tracer condition for preventive services for women (Kessner *et al.* 1977). It causes 2000 deaths in the UK per annum and there is a screening test, the cervical smear. The cervical cytology programme in a practice is a good performance indicator. An audit of cervical cytology will not only tell a great deal about the cervical cytology programme, but also the practice team's attitudes to prevention, and the effectiveness of the organization in delivering care in the preventive area.

Developing a practice policy

All members of the practice team involved in preventive care for women should meet to agree an appropriate policy. The discussion might usefully start with a statement of aims, such as:

This practice aims to:

1. Inform the patients about prevention, and to deal with their concerns regarding this.
2. Prevent the following conditions:
   (a) Coronary artery disease
   (b) Lung cancer
   (c) Obesity
   (d) Unwanted pregnancy
   (e) Sexually transmitted diseases
   (f) Breast cancer
   (g) Cervical cancer
   (h) Menopausal problems

The next step is for the practice to agree a *management plan* for its well-women's clinic. This might look something like this:

1. Women between the ages of 25 and 64 years should be invited every 3 or 5 years to attend the well-women's clinic (this age range and frequency of attendance should be adapted to local circumstances).
2. Patients' concerns regarding their health should be attended to.
3. Patients should be informed about preventive care available.
4. Height and weight should be measured and Body Mass Index calculated (weight/height^2).
5. Smoking, drug taking, alcohol intake, diet, and exercise should be discussed and appropriate advice given.
6. Breasts should be examined and if the woman is between the ages of 50 and 64 years the National Mammography programme discussed.
7. A cervical smear should be performed if necessary.

8. If the woman is over 40 she should be asked about any problems relating to the menopause and consideration should be given to hormone replacement therapy.

Developing standards, i.e. criteria for assessment and levels of performance

It is not reasonable to review every aspect of the management in a well-women's clinic and it is best to start simply:

Basic criteria for assessing a well-women's clinic

1. A woman aged between 25 and 64 years should attend the well-women's clinic every 3 or 5 years.
2. At each attendance the agreed management plan should be carried out.

Once simple attendance has been examined, it is likely that the practice would want to look further at the quality of care in the clinic. As has been discussed before, cervical cancer is a good tracer condition for preventive services for women.

Suggested criteria for assessing a cervical cancer screening programme

1. A woman with an intact uterus, between the ages of 25 and 64 years, should have a cervical smear every 5 years.
2. The cervical smear taken should be adequate.
3. An abnormal cervical smear should have appropriate follow-up.

Once the group has decided on criteria it must decide what levels of performance it wishes to attain with respect to each of these criteria.

Suggested targets for a well-women's clinic

1. That 80 per cent of women between the ages of 25 and 64 years attend the well-women's clinic.
2. That 80 per cent of those attending should have the agreed management plan adhered to.

Suggested targets for cervical screening

1. That 80 per cent of women who have not had a hysterectomy should have had an adequate cervical smear within 5 years.
2. That not more than 5 per cent of the cervical cytology specimens should be returned by the laboratory as 'inadequate'.

3. That all patients with severe abnormalities and 90 per cent of those with mild or moderate abnormalities should be followed-up to ensure appropriate management.

Clearly, one of the other items in the management plan could have been reviewed rather than cervical cytology. Indeed, the criteria suggested here are all very basic. Once a practice is achieving them comfortably then perhaps it is time to develop others, for example that all women should understand the practice's policy on hormone replacement therapy and be able to make an informed choice about it. This would be more of a challenge, both to perform and to assess.

Collecting and analysing the data

If the practice is computerized it is very likely that the software contains space, not only for entering the cervical smear status, but also for recording whether the patient has had a well-person check. If these provisions have been used then a large part of the audit can be done very quickly (Shepherd 1989; Lawrence *et al.* 1990).

By 1990 only 50 per cent of practices had a computer, so many still require manual procedures—and with the numbers involved it is likely that a sampling procedure will be required (in which case read Chapter 6, to ensure that your sample is adequate and unbiased).

A simple recording document is shown in Table 9.6 on which the well-woman clinic and cervical cytology data can be entered from the notes of each patient in the sample.

For recording the proportion of cervical smears which were adequate a note search will not suffice, as it is unlikely that a record will be kept of an inadequate

Table 9.6 *Record sheet for well-woman clinic and cervical cytology data*

	Patient number					
Data	1	2	3	4	5	6
Age						
Date last seen in well-woman clinic						
Management plan complete (yes/no?)						
Hysterectomy (yes/no?)						
Date of last cervical smear						
Place of last cervical smear						
Result (normal/abnormal?)						
If abnormal, degree (moderate/severe?)						
If abnormal followed up (yes/no?)						

smear if this has been followed-up by an adequate one. This information could be collected directly from the laboratory.

Once this has been done the results of the audit can be presented to the practice team in the form of a simple table (Table 9.7).

Evaluating the data and managing change

It is likely that the following problems will be found (among others):

1. Poor recording of information in the notes.
2. Poor attendance at well-women clinic, especially in socially deprived areas.
3. Inefficient and ineffective call and recall systems.
4. Poor adherence to agreed management plans, especially if some professionals feel ambivalent about them or if the time available is inadequate.
5. Too many inadequate cervical smears.

At the meeting to discuss the results it should be pointed out how much effort had to be expended in tracking information which should have been in the notes. This should make it apparent to all members of the team how important good recording of information is.

Poor attendance may reflect either the practice's method of invitation, or a reluctance by women to take up the invitation. The practice should satisfy itself that the invitation system is foolproof (perhaps by sending invitations and reminders, and thereafter tagging the notes for an opportunistic approach). Or perhaps the practice should review whether the form of service being offered is appropriate, especially in socially deprived areas: the time, structure, location, staffing, or service of the clinic may need to be reviewed.

The call and recall should be the responsibility of a named person and should be constantly updated. All pertinent information should be channelled through that person, for example, new registration, transfers out, women having

Table 9.7 *Results of audit of well-women's clinic*

Item	Target (%)
Percentage of women aged 25–64 years who attended clinic in the last 3 or 5 years	80%
Percentage of women attending clinic who had management plan adhered to	80%
Percentage of women with intact uterus who have had an adequate cervical smear in past 5 years	80%
Percentage of smears taken which were inadequate	5%
Percentage of women with severe dyskaryosis who have been followed up	100%

hysterectomies. Much will probably be learned by the group from examination in detail of certain patients for whom recall has failed. In particular, the case of any patient found to have cervical pathology which was not followed up could form the basis of a critical incident audit.

If it is found that the management plans are not being carried out the group should discuss this and perhaps new plans should be agreed, educational input arranged, or more time allocated to the clinic.

Finally, if it is found that too many cervical smears are inadequate discussions should be held with the laboratory to illuminate the problem prior to the audit review meeting. Refresher courses in technique or changes in equipment, for example new specula or cervical brushes, may be needed.

Repeating the audit cycle

Once these changes have been agreed the exercise in data collection and examination should be repeated after a period of 6–12 months to see if results have improved. To be effective the audit cycle should be constantly repeated and once the group is consistently achieving its targets, more sophisticated criteria may be adopted.

Examples

A study undertaken by the author shows the benefit of audit in raising cervical cytology uptake. It was carried out in a new town practice of 10 000 patients (Pierce *et al.* 1989). A total of 1232 women between the ages of 35 and 60 years were identified. From examination of the notes 650 women were found to have had a cervical smear within the past 5 years and 166 had had a hysterectomy.

The practice was achieving a rate of $\dfrac{650}{(1232 - 166)} \times 100 = 64\%$

The 416 women who needed to be invited for a smear were allocated to three groups: one group had a letter, the second had the notes tagged, and the third had no special intervention. During the next year 32 per cent and 27 per cent of the patients in the two intervention groups had a cervical smear, but only 15 per cent of the control group. By then the practice had achieved a 75 per cent performance level.

The practice then decided that, if a woman was due for a cervical smear, a letter of invitation would be sent followed up by a reminder; and the woman's notes would be tagged so that any doctor consulting would be reminded to suggest that she should have a cervical smear done. Following this, a third data collection exercise showed an achieved level of performance of 85 per cent. This has been sustained since then.

A second example is a rather different type of audit. This was an audit cycle performed by members of the Royal College of General Practitioners Vale of

Trent Faculty between 1985 and 1988 (Wilson 1990). A large group of practices did a retrospective audit on 100 sets of notes in 1985 and again in 1988. The practices were asked about their policy with regard to cervical cytology prior to each audit. This audit showed changes in policy and improvements in performance from 1985 to 1988.

REFERENCES

Curtis Jenkins, G. H., Collins, C., and Andrew, S. (1978). Developmental Surveillance in General Practice. *British Medical Journal*, **1**, 1537–40.

Department of Health and Welsh Office. (1989). *General Practice in the National Health Service. A new contract*. Department of Health and the Welsh Office, London.

Hall, D. M. B., Hill, P., and Elliman, D. (1990). *The child surveillance handbook, 1990*. Radcliffe Medical Press, Oxford.

Hall, D. M. B. (ed.) (1992). *Health for all children (2nd edn)*. Oxford University Press.

Holland, W. W. and Stewart, S. (1990). *Screening in health care*. London: Nuffield Provincial Hospitals Trust.

Kessner, D. M., Kalth, C. E., and Singer, J. (1977). Assessing health quality — the case for tracers. *New England Journal of Medicine*, **288**, 189–94.

Lawrence, M., Coulter, A., and Jones, L. (1990). A total audit of preventive procedures in 45 practices caring for 430,000 patients. *British Medical Journal*, **300** (6738), 1501–3.

Pierce, M., Lundy, S., Palanisamy, A., Winning, S., and King, J. (1989). Prospective randomised controlled trial of methods of call and recall for cervical cytology. *British Medical Journal*, **299** (6692), 160–2.

Rossdale, M., Clark, C., and James, J. (1986). Improved health care delivery in an inner city well baby clinic run by general practitioners. *Journal of the Royal College of General Practitioners*, **36**, 512–13.

Royal College of General Practitioners. (1982). *Healthier children — thinking prevention*. Report from General Practice 22. Royal College of General Practitioners, London.

Sheldon Report. (1967). Sub committee of Standing Medical Advisory Committee Child Welfare Centres Report (Chairman W. Sheldon). HMSO, London.

Shepherd, S. (1989). Audit for all — but how? *The Practitioner*, **233**, 1028–31.

UK Trial of early detection of breast cancer. (1988). First results on mortality reduction in UK trial of early detection of breast cancer. *Lancet*, **2**, 411–16.

Wilson, A. (1990). Cervical cytology in the Vale of Trent Faculty of Royal College of General Practitioners 1985–8. *British Medical Journal*, **300**, 376–8.

10 Preventive care: cardiovascular disease

Andrew Farmer

CHOOSING THE TOPIC

Cardiovascular diseases are the most common cause of premature death in the UK. Heart disease leads to disability and a restricted life-style for those suffering from angina and heart failure. The economic cost of treating established heart disease is high. Intensive care for those suffering myocardial infarction is expensive, new drugs such as streptokinase offer improved survival but at great cost, and coronary artery bypass grafting is an increasingly common procedure. Developing a coherent strategy for the prevention of cardiovascular disease has been a priority of many groups, including the government, royal colleges, and district and regional health authorities.

The effectiveness of different strategies for the detection and management of risk factors for cardiovascular disease remain unproven. One strategy is to offer patients a routine blood pressure check and discuss other risk factors as part of a consultation for other matters. Health checks carried out by nurses have also been advocated as a low cost, low technology means of achieving the objective of a reduction in cardiovascular disease (Fullard *et al.* 1987). Critics of this approach have pointed out that such strategies only reach those least in need of the care (Waller *et al.* 1990), and that the costs involved in implementing a successful strategy have been seriously underestimated (Imperial Cancer Research Fund OXCHECK Group 1991).

Offering help to motivated individuals at risk of heart disease is undoubtedly of benefit. Brief advice from general practitioners is successful in motivating individuals to stop smoking (Russell *et al.* 1979), and treatment of mild hypertension is successful in reducing the incidence of stroke, and possibly also cardiac events (Medical Research Council Working Party 1985; Collins *et al.* 1990). However, the extra work that may be required to contact those individuals who are not motivated to stop smoking or lose weight may reduce the resources available for the care of those with other problems. These potential difficulties make it important that any attempt to develop systematic identification and management of cardiovascular risk factors should be carefully monitored for both the results and the workload generated.

Any attempts to detect and manage risk factors for cardiovascular disease need to be planned systematically by all members of the team. Such a programme must incorporate some form of performance review in order to assess whether it is effective. Many studies have highlighted deficiencies in the care of patients with risk factors for cardiovascular disease. They have shown poor initial assessment of individuals, inadequate recording of risk factors, and a failure to achieve adequate control of high blood pressure (Stern 1986; Smith *et al.* 1990). Many of the deficiencies highlighted were due to deficiencies of organization and lack of systematic care, rather than to any deficiencies in knowledge or skills.

DEVELOPING A PLAN OF CARE

Earlier chapters have already stressed the possibility of entering the audit cycle at any point. Most examples of audits of cardiovascular disease begin either with collecting data or with trying to develop a plan of care.

Developing a plan of care involves members of the practice in considering scientific evidence about the interventions proposed, the local availability of resources, and the preferences of the team members involved in providing care.

An example of a plan for the care of hypertensive patients is shown in Fig. 10.1. Different plans may emerge in time—parts of the protocol may involve an excessive workload, or further evidence may emerge that requires some parts to be dropped and others to be modified or added to. Over the past few years there has been an increased understanding of the need for the integrated management of risk factors for cardiovascular disease. Other items reflect personal preferences, such as the requirement for two yearly assessment of renal function and fundal examination to be carried out.

The care plan is the source from which criteria for audit can be developed.

CRITERIA FOR AUDIT

There are so many aspects of cardiovascular disease that can be audited that it is often good to start with easier ones and develop the audit as the team becomes more competent. Criteria are conventionally divided into those based on the organization and facilities available (structure), the interventions that are actually made (process), and the end results of interventions such as control of blood pressure (intermediate outcome) or number of heart attacks (outcome).

Ideally a criterion is an objective of care for which every practice would wish to achieve a level of performance of 100 per cent. Most target standards represent a compromise because either the practice has felt unable to set a level of performance of 100 per cent, or the criterion does not state precisely the objectives of care for every patient in the group (for instance, there may well be hypertensives for whom it might be inappropriate to aim for a diastolic blood pressure less than 90 mmHg). A purely objective approach to care also excludes the wider consideration of factors that might affect the appropriateness of interventions for individual patients.

Management for established hypertensives under 70 years

Measurement

Blood pressures should be measured with the patient in a sitting position with the forearm supported at the level of the chest. The reading should be taken to the nearest 2 mmHg.

Blood pressure control

Blood pressure should be maintained below 160/90. If this is not possible, the target pressure should be stated in the notes.

End organ damage

Examination of fundi and peripheral pulses and assessment of renal function should be made every 2 years. An electrocardiogram should be taken 5 yearly.

Risk factor management

1. Help should be given to achieve an ideal weight.

2. Help should be given to stop smoking.

3. Serum cholesterol should be measured 5 yearly. The level should be under 6.5 mm/l.

4. Alcohol intake should be 20 units or less for men and 14 units or less for women.

Drug therapy

1. Drugs used should be thiazides, β-blockers, calcium antagonists or ACE inhibitors, singly or in appropriate combinations.

2. Side-effects and compliance should be assessed at each visit. Action should be taken to minimize side-effects and maximize compliance in all cases.

Education

Patients should be regularly reminded of the nature of hypertension, the reason for treatment, the importance of other risk factors, and be involved in their own care.

Follow-up

1. Patients with treated blood pressure above 160/90 or those with other risk factors needing treatment, side-effects or poor compliance should be seen 3-monthly. Otherwise follow up 6 monthly.

2. Referral to hospital should be made if the target pressure is not achieved with 3 drugs despite good compliance, or if there is a possibility of secondary hypertension.

3. Stopping treatment should be considered if pressure is < 90 mmHg on one drug, if there is a significant reduction in weight or alcohol intake, or if disadvantages of treatment outweigh advantages.

4. A list of patients receiving treatment for hypertension should be available and up to date. An annual check should be made to identify and follow up defaulters.

Fig. 10.1 An example management plan for care of hypertensive patients.

Structure

Items of structure offer an easy starting point for examining the care provided within a practice. Examples include:

1. Is there a systematic recording method? One example is the use of structured record cards from which information about care can easily be retrieved; another would be a policy for uniform recording of blood pressures, drugs, and cardiovascular risk factors on a computer.
2. Is there a call/recall method? This may be a sophisticated method of sending postal reminders to patients, or a means of adding reminders to the clinical notes in order to identify patients attending for other problems.
3. Are the sphygmomanometers regularly checked? Is there a person with responsibility for seeing that the machines are serviced?
4. Does the practice have an ECG machine available?
5. Is there a register of hypertensive patients? Are the criteria for inclusion in the register defined? Are hypertensives on treatment clearly distinguished from those who are borderline hypertensives requiring regular review?

Process

The contents of the medical record are easily examined and therefore provide an accessible and convenient basis for an audit of the detection of risk factors for cardiovascular disease.

1. Has the blood pressure been recorded in the past year?
2. Has the smoking habit been recorded?
3. Has the alcohol intake been recorded?
4. Has the serum cholesterol been recorded?
5. Has the family history been recorded?
6. Has the weight been recorded?
7. Has the patient been advised about diet?
8. Has the patient been offered advice about giving up smoking?
9. Is the current medication identifiable from the medical records?
10. Was the blood pressure recorded at least three times before treatment was initiated?

Outcome

The most valuable measures of the care provided are those dealing with outcomes important to patients. Some outcomes, such as the control of blood pressure or serum cholesterol are intermediate measures. Intermediate measures are only important in so far as they reflect final outcomes, such as morbidity and mortality. Examples include:

1. Is the diastolic blood pressure less than 90 mmHg?

2. Is the patient a smoker?
3. Is the quality of life impaired by treatment?
4. Is the patient experiencing drug related side-effects?
5. Has the patient had a stroke?
6. Has the patient had a heart attack?

COLLECTING THE DATA

Some data collection, particularly regarding structure, may require very little effort. A meeting of the primary health care team can work through a checklist looking at the care provided, identifying areas that are already covered, and highlighting deficiencies. Most audit, particularly of process or outcome, will require systematic data collection. Medical records may provide the most ready source of such information, but occasionally other systems may have to be set up to record relevant information.

Problems that need to be resolved before starting an audit include:

1. How is the group forming the denominator for the audit to be defined? All those with serum cholesterols over 6.5 mmol/l on any occasion; those on drug treatment; those attending a practice clinic?
2. What time period should the audit cover?
3. How precisely are the criteria for audit defined? Would a comment on obesity be sufficient to constitute a record of weight?
4. Is the pro forma for data collection drawn up satisfactorily?

Increasingly, data collection is being carried out using computers. This enables automatic repetitive searches to be carried out with minimal effort, and the performance of practices collated and used in feedback (Lawrence *et al*. 1990).

Many medical record audits are now carried out by nurses or clerical staff rather than doctors. The criteria need to be developed by a team involving those delivering the care (including doctors and nurses) and those providing back-up and collecting the data (practice clerical and reception staff). The criteria developed are then shared by the team, which becomes committed to implementing any changes that may be required. Information collected as a chore by a clerk who had no involvement in developing the audit is unlikely to be accurate.

Data that is relatively easy to collect (often structure and process) may be less informative than data that is more difficult to collect (often outcome measures). First, many criteria based on structure or process may have little relationship to outcome. A practice may accurately record the smoking habit of all their hypertensives, but offer no advice about stopping smoking. Secondly, some data that is fairly easy to collect (for example the number of strokes or heart attacks) may be relatively rare events and therefore their rate may vary randomly in a small population. As a practice becomes more experienced in audit there is increased satisfaction from systematically looking at aspects of care that are more difficult to measure but are more important to patients, such as the quality of life and the incidence of side-effects.

EVALUATION AND MAKING CHANGES

Perhaps the most important area of all is in making changes. Performance review is primarily an educational process rather than a means of justifying performance. The results of the audit should allow an opportunity to reflect on the gap between aspiration and performance and the barriers to change. This should then be followed by an agreement on action to achieve change, agreement on a timetable, and an agreement to review progress.

The type of audits discussed for the care of cardiovascular disease lend themselves to group discussion within the practice. Results need to be disseminated within the practice. Those involved in care or audit should have a chance to review the criteria and discuss the results in order to remain committed to improving the standards of care. Deficiencies that are revealed may lead to changes for the receptionists (changes in the call and recall of patients) or for the medical staff (changing the use of drugs or tighter control of blood pressure): alternatively criteria which were felt to be unreasonable may be changed after discussion.

The audit may show that relevant information was not present in the notes. What is not written down cannot be retrieved. In order to improve patient care through auditing the notes it may be necessary to agree on systematic data recording. Structured record cards are one way of achieving this.

Audit also leads to the identification of educational needs. Staff may request extra training in the use of recall systems on the practice computer, medical staff may feel the need for more information about the indication for using new drugs. If the set targets are achieved, then further review may be put off for some time and another area of care examined.

AN EXAMPLE OF AUDIT OF PROCESS

Oxford rent-an-audit

The Oxford Prevention of Heart Attack and Stroke project (Fullard *et al.* 1984, 1987) was set up following a series of reports that described the scope for preventive activities in primary care. One of the reports concluded 'about half of all strokes and a quarter of all deaths from coronary heart disease in people under the age 70 are probably preventable by the application of existing knowledge' (Royal College of General Practitioners 1981).

In this project the practice reception staff checked the notes of patients aged 35–64 years attending the surgery. If the patient had not had a recent health check then a prompt card was placed in the notes. The patients were then encouraged by the doctor and reception staff to take up the offer of a health check with the practice nurse.

The practice nurses carrying out the checks gave advice about stopping smoking, weight reduction, improved diet, and increasing exercise. The information was recorded on a structured record card (Fig. 10.2) and filed in the patient's notes.

Clearly it was necessary to assess the effect of the intervention on the recording of cardiovascular risk factors. The three criteria chosen for the audit were that there should be records of smoking habit, weight, and blood pressure in the patients' notes. The method chosen for the audit was a 10 per cent sample of the notes of patients aged 35–64 years. For the purpose of the project the data collection was carried out by a team of trained audit clerks. Patients were identified using the age-sex register held by the practice. For each audit a date was chosen before which all entries were ignored. The precise criteria chosen were fairly generous, for instance any mention of weight such as a comment 'obese' was considered acceptable.

An initial audit was carried out and the results fed back to practices along with information about the performance of other practices. Over a period of two years, help was offered to improve the systems established. With this approach the recording of blood pressure, smoking habit, and weight increased dramatically (Fig. 10.3).

The rolling audit

Prompted by the need to have continuing information about its prevention activities, the author's practice had set up a similar audit and coined the phase 'rolling audit'. Criteria for the recording of preventive procedures were developed by a clerical staff member and trainee and agreed by the practice team: they varied with age band (men aged 35–70 years; women aged 16–24, 25–34, 35–40, and 41–70 years; children aged 2–15 years).

Criteria relating to cardiovascular disease prevention are assessed in the age band 35–70 years. They are 'Had the blood pressure been recorded in the past five years?, is there a record of smoking?, is there a record of alcohol intake?, is the Body Mass Index (BMI) recorded?'. Each year a 10 per cent sample of records for each age/sex group is identified and the notes examined by the clerical staff member; the sample was originally identified from the age/sex register, now from a computer printout.

The results are presented annually at the practice meeting including doctors, nurses, and receptionists. Some of the results are shown in Fig. 10.4. These results show a steady increase in the recording of alcohol intake for men, but a plateau in the increase in blood pressure and smoking recording in 1987

Health summary

Female

Name

Date of birth		SMWD		No.	

Own occupation
Partner's occupation

Date	Date	Date	
1st blood pressure	2nd blood pressure	3rd blood pressure	Mean if applicable

Weight	Ideal weight		Height	

Smoker	Cigarettes	Pipe	Since 19
Non-smoker	Never	Stopped 19	

Family history of stroke or heart attack

Diabetes	Yes	Insulin	OHD	Diet
	No			

Oral contraception years of use	Current	Past	Never

IUD	Current	Past	Parity

Last cervical smear	Date	Result

Rubella	Immune	Yes	No	Date
	Vaccination	Yes	No	Date

Date of tetanus	1st	2nd	3rd	Booster

Urine date	Protein	Sugar

Alcohol

Allergies

Notes/Past operations

Fig. 10.2 Patient record card.

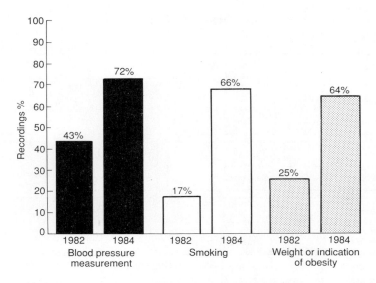

Fig. 10.3   Recordings in the previous five years on 1 April 1982 and 11 June 1984, based on a 10 per cent sample of the records of patients aged 35−64 years (Fullard *et al.* 1984).

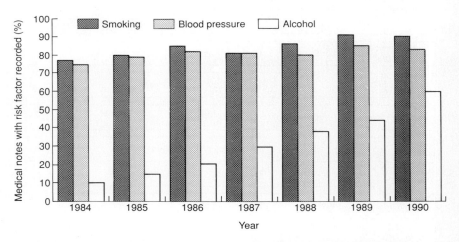

Fig. 10.4   Percentage of medical notes with risk factors recorded (35−70 years).

followed by a further rise. This illustrates the value of changing in response to results, because the 1987 results stimulated a new prompt card stuck on to the front of the notes—following which recording rates again increased. Another area of discussion arising from the audit has been the role of nurses in opportunistic screening.

The widespread adoption of health checks demonstrates the effectiveness of using simple measures that can give encouragement, together with a clearly defined and simple strategy that can be easily adapted to the circumstances of different practices. The main criticisms levelled at these audits of process are firstly that they do not define individuals with adverse risks with a view to specific management follow-up: and that they provide no measure of success in the management of risk factors in individuals. For this it is necessary to audit (intermediate) outcome.

AN AUDIT OF INTERMEDIATE OUTCOME

Hypertension management project

The hypertension management project was undertaken to look at the follow up offered to those identified with, and treated for, raised blood pressure. In particular it was aimed at the blood pressure control achieved, the identification and management of risk factors, the education offered to patients and the side-effects experienced by patients.

Eight practices agreed to be involved in the project. A series of criteria were developed and used as the basis for an audit.

Criteria of structure

1. Is there a protocol for screening and management of hypertension?
2. Are practice nurses involved in screening, assessment, and education?
3. Is there a systematic follow-up system for defaulters?

Criteria of process

1. Is there a recording of smoking habit, weight, cholesterol, and alcohol intake in the past five years?
2. Has the patient been reviewed in the past year?
3. Was the blood pressure measured to 2 mmHg?

Criteria of outcome

1. Is the blood pressure less than 160/90?
2. Did the patient recall advice about smoking, diet, and alcohol intake?

The notes of hypertensive patients were identified from disease indexes or from repeat medication registers. An audit of these notes was then carried out using either the notes of all hypertensive patients aged 21–64 years, or a sample of at least 100 notes.

Patients' views and opinions of their care were also gathered using a series of questions and a standard health questionnaire.

The results were then correlated for all the practices and fed back to meetings of the whole primary health care team including doctors, nurses, practice managers, and often reception staff. Each practice received its own results together with the aggregated results of the other practices. The main findings were that:

1. The level of risk factor recording varied widely between practices.
2. Some practices had a number of hypertensives on treatment with no record of blood pressure in the past year.
3. Some practices were recording six or more blood pressures each year, even though the level had been reduced to normal.

Several practices took measures to bring about change.

1. One practice identified those with no blood pressure recorded in the previous year and invited them to a nurse run clinic.
2. One practice invited all those on treatment to a nurse clinic to identify and offer help to those with adverse risk factors.
3. One practice employed a clerk to go through notes, extracting information about risk factors, writing them on the summary card and highlighting missing data.

This is an example of a group project—but a similar exercise could be carried out by a single practice. There might be even more incentive for a practice to change because of the increased feelings of ownership through devising its own audit.

SUMMARY

The detection and management of risk factors for cardiovascular disease is one of the most important public health problems facing the health service. A systematic approach to management requires that plans of care be based on realistic assessments of scientific evidence, and take account of the workload involved.

Simple criteria for care, measuring aspects of structure, process and outcome, are easily drawn up. With a little planning, data to measure the level of performance for these criteria can be collected and used as part of a performance review process. Change in unlikely to take place unless the whole practice feels involved in the process.

ACKNOWLEDGEMENTS

I would like to acknowledge the work of Andrew Markus, Ken Burch, and John Derry in developing the 'rolling audit'. I would also like to acknowledge the work of Peter Rose in developing the hypertension management project.

REFERENCES

Collins, R., Peto, R., MacMahon, S., Hebert, P., Fiebach, N. H., Eberlein, K. A. *et al.* (1990). Blood pressure, stroke, and coronary heart disease. Part 2. *Lancet*, **335**, 827–38.

Fullard, E., Fowler, G., and Gray, J. A. M. (1984). Facilitating prevention in primary care. *British Medical Journal*, **289**, 1585–7.

Fullard, E., Fowler, G., and Gray, J. A. M. (1987). Promoting prevention in primary care: controlled trial of low technology, low cost approach. *British Medical Journal*, **294**, 1080–2.

Imperial Cancer Research Fund OXCHECK Study Group. (1991). Prevalence of risk factors for heart disease in OXCHECK trial: implications for screening in primary care. *British Medical Journal*, **302**, 1057–60.

Lawrence, M. S., Coulter, A., and Jones, L. (1990). A total audit of preventive procedures in 45 practices caring for 430,000 patients. *British Medical Journal*, **300**, 1501–3.

Medical Research Council Working Party. (1985). MRC trial of treatment of mild hypertension: principal results. *British Medical Journal*, **291**, 97–104.

Royal College of General Practitioners. (1981). *Prevention of arterial disease in general practice*. RCGP, London.

Russell, M. A. H., Wilson, C., Taylor, C., and Baker, C. D. Effect of general practitioners' advice against smoking. *British Medical Journal*, **2**, 231–5.

Smith, W. C. S., Lee, A. J., Crombie, I. K., and Tunstall-Pedoe, H. (1990). Control of blood pressure in Scotland: the rule of halves. *British Medical Journal*, **300**, 981–3.

Stern, D. Management of hypertension in twelve Oxfordshire general practices. (1986). *Journal of the Royal College of General Practitioners*, **36**, 549–51.

Waller, D., Agass, M., Mant, D., Coulter, A., Fuller, A., and Jones, L. (1990). Health checks in general practice: another example of inverse care? *British Medical Journal*, **300**, 1115–18.

11 Chronic disease management

John Hasler

Chronic disease is one of the key areas for audit in primary health care, for several reasons. It uses up a substantial amount of resources, both in time and money; it is often possible to draw conclusions about outcome from the examination of process, by reference to published evidence; some of the parameters are easily measurable (for example, blood pressure levels, blood glucose measurements, serum phenytoin measurement, and peak flow rates); the data are easily extractable, provided that the manual or electronic records systems are designed appropriately; chronic diseases are frequently supervised by nurses as well as doctors and therefore it is possible to audit team care rather than simply medical care.

In this section we will examine two common chronic diseases, although the principles are the same for most chronic diseases and readers should constantly consider the applicability of the messages to other long-term conditions in which they have an interest.

DIABETES MELLITUS

Choosing the topic

Diabetes has been chosen as an example for a number of reasons. It is a relatively common problem, affecting between 1 and 2 per cent of the population, which means that each general practitioner in the UK will have on average between 20 and 40 diabetic patients, of whom only a minority will be insulin dependent. It has a significant number of potential complications including blindness, increased atherosclerosis, renal disease, and neuropathy: there is increasing evidence that good glucose control and management of other risk factors will reduce these risks. Diabetes uses up a significant amount of NHS resources, both in hospital and general practice. Many general practitioners are still somewhat reluctant to take over the routine care of diabetic patients, and auditing this care is one way to improve their skill and confidence, whilst ensuring that resources are used in the most effective way.

Studies have shown that appropriate general practice care can reduce hospital admissions and referrals (Cox 1983) and that it can be as good as hospital care (Singh *et al.* 1984). Conversely, the delivery of care can also be disorganized and ineffective (Hayes and Harries 1984).

Developing a plan for care and criteria for audit

There is a whole range of items that need to be managed and evaluated. They fall into several categories.

1. Measurements.
   The most important of these is blood glucose. Glycosylated haemoglobin is an important indicator of long-term control, especially for patients managed on insulin, but in some areas the latter measurements are not routinely available, and fructosamine levels may have to be accepted instead. Other important measurements are visual acuity, blood pressure, weight, urine tests for glucose and protein, lipid levels, and renal function.
2. Clinical examination.
   In addition to these measurements other examinations that should be carried out on a regular basis include examination of the retinae and feet.
3. Patient education.
   In no chronic disease is patient education of more importance. Subjects include management of illness and emergencies, adjustment of insulin dosages, diet (preferably taught by a dietician), care of the feet (preferably by a chiropodist), and testing urine or blood for glucose. It is helpful if patients are advised to join the British Diabetic Association, which will provide them with helpful leaflets: car drivers also need to be advised to inform the licensing authority.

Records

Whilst it would be time-consuming to examine all these activities every time diabetic care is audited, it is important that as far as possible comprehensive data are collected regularly. This requires a specially designed flow sheet in the manual records (Fig. 11.1) or a computerized data collection system. For managing care, flow sheets also remind doctors and nurses what has been agreed in the protocol. For assessing care they must be created in such a way that an audit clerk without detailed medical knowledge can extract the information.

Agreeing criteria and target levels of performance

There is always a problem in deciding what target standards a practice wishes to set when auditing diabetic care. Some items are not controversial, such as the need to check a diabetic patient's eyes regularly; but different doctors have different views about what level of fasting blood sugar indicates good or acceptable diabetic control.

The use of criteria and levels of performance helps greatly in this situation. For example, with regard to fasting blood glucose (FBG) the practice may choose to examine whether patients have FBG less 10 and less than 8, and then set different target levels of performance for the two measurements. The more

DIABETIC CARD

Name ....

Address ....

....

....

Date of birth ....

Date of Diagnosis ....

General practitioner ....

	BDA	Prescription	Sugar		DVLC	Target weight
			Hypos	Insurance		

Presentation
Diabetic summary

Other medical history

Family history

Smoking

Lipids

Urea

HbA,C

Date	Blood sugar	Blood pressure	Urine S/P/K	Weight	Visual activity L R	Fundi	Feet	Pulses	Treatment	Comments	Next appointment

Fig. 11.1 Data record card for diabetes.

precisely defined the criterion, the more meaningful will be the resulting target—thus 'fasting blood glucose should be less than 8 in patients aged under 65 years and less than 10 in patients over 65 years', may be more rigorous than 'FBG should be less than 10' and more achievable than 'FBG should be less than 8'.

It is usually helpful to start assessing criteria of structure, then to move on to process, and finally to use criteria of (intermediate) outcome. This is because, although outcome audit is the ideal, structure and process are easier to measure, and it is almost always better to start simply. Examples of criteria which practices may wish to use are given in Table 11.1. Having agreed the criteria to be measured, it will be necessary for the practice to set a target level of performance. In many cases there is no argument and the level should be 100 per cent, especially for items of structure. For most items of process too, the level of performance is likely to be set high. For outcome measures there will be more debate and need to refer to the literature, and targets will probably be set with reference to currently achieved levels.

Collecting the data

Identification

In these days of ubiquitous computers it is increasingly common to find that diabetic patients are identified electronically. Most of them will have been identified initially through the repeat prescribing of drugs which are specific for diabetes. That leaves those diabetic patients who are maintained on diet alone: gradually these should be found as they attend for periodic supervision.

A problem with computer data storage is the variety of codes that may be used for diabetes. For audit purposes just three categories are needed—those on diet control, taking oral therapy, and using insulin.

Practices still without computerized disease registers can manage perfectly well with manual ones made up either as a card index or a loose-leaf book: it is important to remember to update it each time a new diabetic patient is identified.

Sampling

For the purposes of auditing, it is important to decide what group of patients should be investigated. Since the management of individual diabetic patients is so important, and there are likely to be only 30 or so per doctor, it will usually be possible to examine the whole group. Certainly, if individual drugs are of interest the appropriate group can probably be looked at in its entirety unless the practice population is very large; and when examining computer held data it will also be feasible to look at the whole group. However, if manual records have to be extracted in a large practice it may be felt necessary to take a sample.

Table 11.1   *Draft criteria for assessment of diabetic care*

Criteria of structure of the practice

1. Is there a register of diabetics?
2. Does it include: (a) insulin treated,
                    (b) oral hypoglycaemics,
                    (c) diet control?
3. Do diabetics comprise between 1 and 2 per cent of the practice population?
4. Is there a diabetic clinic? If not, is there another systematic method of care?
5. Is the practice nurse involved in the management of diabetics?
6. Are there arrangements to review those who cannot get to surgery?
7. Is there a written management protocol?

Criteria of process and (intermediate) outcome

1. Is the patient under: (a) hospital care?
                         (b) general practitioner care?
                         (c) shared care?
2. Is the patient on the practice recall system?
3. Was the patient seen for diabetic review in the past year?
4. Has the blood pressure been measured in the past year?
   (a) If so was the diastolic blood pressure < 100 mmHg?
   (b) If so was the diastolic blood pressure < 90 mmHg?
5. Has the fasting glucose been measured in the past year?
   (a) If so, was the glucose < 10mmol/l?
   (b) Was the glucose < 8mmol/l?
6. Has the HbA1C or fructosamine been measured in the past year?
   (a) If so, was HbA1C < 10% or fructosamine < 300μmol/l?
7. Has the cholesterol level been measured in the past five years?
   (a) If so, was the last cholesterol level < 8mmol/1?
   (b) Was the last cholesterol level < 6.5mmol/1?
8. Has the blood urea/creatinine been measured in the last five years?
   (a) If so, was it normal?
9. Has the urine been checked for proteinurea in the past year?
   (a) If so, was it negative?
10. Is there a smoking record in the notes?
    (a) If so, is the patient a smoker?
11. Have the fundi been examined in the past year?
    (a) If so, were they normal?
12. Has the visual acuity been measured in the past year?
    (a) If so, was it normal?
13. Have the feet been examined in the past year?
    (a) If so, was the circulation normal?
    (b) Was the sensation normal?
14. Has the weight been measured in the past year?
    (a) Was the Body Mass Index (BMI) < 30?
    (b) Was the BMI < 25?
15. Has the patient been advised to join the British Diabetic Association?
16. Has management of hypoglycaemia been explained?

Whilst selection does not have to be done as scrupulously as it would for a research project, it is, nevertheless, important to make sure that it is reasonably random (see p. 61).

If a variety of doctors are involved in diabetic care, ideally they should be identified as part of the data collection, so that comparative analyses can be done. Since each doctor usually cares for less than 30 diabetic patients, an analysis at this level will require all patients to be in the sample.

Staff involvement

If the audit criteria are clearly identified and the data clearly shown in the computer or the records, then most of the analyses can be done by clerical staff. The doctors and nurses need to agree the criteria (for example Table 11.1), they or a clerical assistant enter the data when the patient attends, and the clerical staff can extract and present it. One of the advantages of running a clinic system for diabetes is that it allows for a clerical assistant to be present to enter information such as glucose levels and blood pressure readings straight into the computer, so saving nurses' and doctors' time.

Evaluating the data

On the whole, unlike with research, most findings should be relatively easy to interpret. Non-attendance, no flow sheets in the notes, empty flow sheets, are easy to understand and the question is how to get everyone to comply with the agreed guidelines. The findings should be presented so that individual doctors and nurses can be identified: it is necessary to ensure that the doctor is the one that looks after the patient and not necessarily the one with whom the patient is registered. Beware of trying to make things too complicated: stick to simple tables that everyone can understand.

Managing change

As time goes by the decisions taken become more detailed. At the start people have to be encouraged to identify patients and record what they are doing. Once they are used to that, it becomes a matter of remembering what to do (for example, check the eyes and feet). Then it is a question not just of doing things but making sure that the results achieved are acceptable (for example, glucose levels, reduction in number of episodes of poor control).

The audit cycle identifies the necessity of not only changing care to achieve targets, but of revisiting the targets themselves in the light of experience. This may involve removing criteria which are no longer regarded as relevant, or toughening criteria which were too easily attained. It may also mean adding targets of outcome to the previous targets of structure and process. Review of management and of target standards needs to be done at a team meeting, with everyone involved present (including any clerks whose job is to collect data). Many practitioners find that it is helpful if the information is presented on an overhead projector: decisions made must be written down and circulated.

The team members need to be encouraged. Do not set the targets too high too quickly. Let them see they are getting results before the goal posts are moved again. Do not leave people out—nurses, dieticians, and clerical staff involved in appointments and audit are just as important as doctors: make them feel involved.

Repeat

From what has just been said and from the earlier examples it is obvious that diabetic audit (like all others) is repetitive, constantly increasing the standard of care given. The key to success is not a snapshop but a circular journey.

EXAMPLE OF AUDIT OF DIABETIC CARE

A practice caring for 6000 patients decided to audit its diabetic care starting in 1988. At the outset only items of process and structure were examined, and some of the results are shown in Table 11.2.

After the 1989 audit a practice meeting was held and the following evaluation and plans were made:

1. Up to date recall is improving but not adequate.
2. A large part of the deficit is in the house bound. *Plan*: involve the district nurse.

Table 11.2 *Identifying and recalling diabetic patients*

Audit				On recall (%)			Up to date (%)			Percentage of registered up to date		
	Registered											
Year	1988	1989	1991	1988	1989	1991	1988	1989	1991	1988	1989	1991
Doctor A	16	15	13	4	6	9	1	4	9	6	26	60
B	34	38	31	26	33	29	14	15	24	41	39	77
C	18	22	24	10	19	21	2	9	18	11	41	75
D	3	6	8	2	4	7	1	3	7	33	50	88
No usual doctor	2	2	0	0	0	0	0	0	0	—	—	—
Totals	73	83	76	43 (58)	62 (75)	66 (87)	18 (43)	31 (50)	58 (88)	25	37	76

3. Considerable defaulting occurs because of difficulty with forward appointments. *Plan*: one receptionist to have special responsibility and send out reminder cards.
4. We need clinical outcome data. *Plan*: the same receptionist to review records according to an agreed list of criteria.

Table 11.2 also shows the continued improvement in recall by 1991. In addition, Table 11.3 shows some of the findings from looking at clinical outcome data in patients on oral hypoglycaemic agents in 1990 and 1991. The printing out of the list of patients from the computer, extraction of the data from medical records, and tabulation of results was done entirely by the receptionist.

The improvement in 1991 was largely due to greater effort following the 1990 audit. Current evaluation and plans following the 1991 audit are:

1. Nine out of 37 patients are still not on recall or are overdue. *Plan*: the receptionist to refer such patients to doctor if found to be overdue in the audit search.
2. Poor glucose control (50 per cent FBG greater than 10). *Plan*: doctors to review carefully at clinic.
3. Poor foot examination. *Plan*: include in the nurses' instead of the doctors' responsibility.

It can be seen from Tables 11.3 and 11.4 that this audit has encouraged and demonstrated improvement in care. Such improvement has not been easy to achieve, and ongoing audit is essential to ensure its maintenance.

Table 11.3 *Continuation of the audit shown in Table 11.2 with clinical data added for patients on oral hypoglycaemics*

	1990	*1991*
Total on oral agents	39	37
On recall	31	33
Overdue	7	5
No blood pressure < 1 year	10	5
Last blood pressure > 100 mmHg	6	2
No glucose < 1 year	6	5
Last glucose > 10mmol/l	14	17
No fundus < 1 year	20	9
No smoking record	6	4
No cholesterol record	17	9
Foot pulses recorded	3	7

ASTHMA

Choosing the topic

Asthma is common and appears to be increasing. There has been evidence over the years of poor care (Speight *et al.* 1983; Levy and Bell 1984), and it can be well managed by a practice nurse. There are 2000 deaths each year. There are many aspects of care amenable to management, and consensus guidelines on management were published on 1990 (British Thoracic Society 1990*a*, *b*).

The application of the audit cycle to asthma care will be demonstrated using the experience of the author's practice as an example.

Developing a plan for care and criteria for audit

Table 11.4 shows the practice's care plan and sets out what the partners and asthma nurse agreed should happen. It was particularly felt that the initial assessment and diagnosis was often sketchy, patient education was poor, and that not enough patients knew what to do when their asthma became unstable.

Records

The record sheet for the intial assessment is shown in Fig. 11.2. All routine asthma care in this practice is provided by a nurse specially trained for this disease and the record makes it easy for everyone to see what has been done.

Table 11.4   *Asthma management protocol*

1. Identify trigger factors (such as exercise or cold air), the effects on work or school and elicit smoking history.
2. Check height, chest shape, and expected Peak Flow Rate (PFR).
3. An initial assessment should include several days PFR recordings at home, response to bronchodilators and an exercise test if indicated.
4. Patients should be given a leaflet, have their aerosol use checked, and be told what to do in an emergency.
5. Smoking (in parents if appropriate) should be strongly discouraged. A peak flow meter should be prescribed.
6. Usual drugs should follow the British Thoracic Society guidelines: inhaled salbutamol, followed by inhaled beclomethasone (or sodium cromoglycate), followed by high dose inhaled beclomethasone.
7. Acute asthma is treated by 60 mg oral prednisolone (30 mg in children) with nebulized salbutamol or terbutaline. Oxygen if appropriate.

Asthma flow card

Trigger factors and other features

Exercise	no	yes		Pollen/grass	no	yes	
Animals	no	yes		Cold air	no	yes	
Dust	no	yes		Food	no	yes	
URTI	no	yes		Laugh	no	yes	
Work effects	no	yes		Emotion	no	yes	
School attendance	no	yes		Family history	no	yes	
Smoking	no	yes		Night cough	no	yes	

Exam   Date ....

Chest shape

Height (cm)	PFR	Expected	Measured

Further PF   Date ....

Response to bronchodilators			Before		After	
Exercise test	Before		After	1.	2.	3.

Home recordings (range and pattern)

Comments

Initial management   Date ....

Leaflet given	no	yes	Aerosol used checked	no	yes	Smoking action	no	yes
PF meter prescribed	no	yes	Emergency instructions	no	yes	On problem list	no	yes

Drugs ....

Fig. 11.2 Asthma record sheet.

Patient education

As with many chronic conditions, patients should be able to manage their own asthma to a large extent. This is reflected in the record sheet where there are spaces for checking items such as whether emergency instructions have been explained and whether a peak flow meter has been prescribed. It is just as important to demonstrate that education and communication have been carried out as it is to demonstrate clinical care.

Audit criteria

The criteria follow from the management plan. The practice agreed that each of the items in the management plan should be carried out in every case!

Collecting the data

Identification

Identifying all the patients is not as easy as it is for diabetes. Although around 6 per cent of the British population suffer from asthma, much goes undetected and some patients only require medication very intermittently. Nevertheless, it should be possible to list all the regular drug takers from the analysis of prescriptions. Those who require some form of emergency intervention, such as nebulized bronchodilators, oral steroids, or hospital admission form an important sub-group of asthma sufferers who warrant special attention. These patients can be identified prospectively and their care audited at intervals, since the aim of every primary care team is to keep these episodes to a minimum: each situation therefore can be examined to determine whether it could have been prevented.

Tables 11.5 and 11.6 show examples of simple data collections relating to patient education and emergency nebulizer use.

Evaluating the data

The findings set out in these examples raise the usual questions about how the shortfall between targets and performance could be reduced.

Interpretation

Regarding patient education, activities were only listed if they were positively recorded in the notes: the number of activities actually performed might have been higher, especially in the case of doctors who did not always have a flow card in the record. Nor do we know how far the 39 patients selected were

Table 11.5 *Asthma audit: patient education*

Doctors

A total of 251 patients were identified with a first diagnosis of asthma in 3 years up to 1 July 1990. These were distributed between doctors: A, 52; B, 37; C, 91; D, 71.

Every sixth record was scrutinized: 39 were available. Only written entries in the notes were accepted. The results were:

Doctor	No.	Leaflet given	Technique checked	Emergency instruction	Referred to nurse
A	7	1	5	2	6
B	2	1	1	1	1
C	18	7	10	7	8
D	12	3	5	3	6
Total	39	12	21	13	21

Nurse

A total of 129 people with asthma had attended the nurse asthma clinic in the first six months of operation in 1989/90.

Nurse	No.	Leaflet given	Technique checked	Emergency instruction
Nurse	129	93	110	118

Table 11.6 *Asthma audit: emergency nebulizer use (Jan 1–June 30 1990)*

TOTAL: The nebulizer was used in emergency on 15 occasions

8 were temporary residents or from another practice.
4 were known not to be taking their drugs.
3 were newly diagnosed.

typical: the numbers were low for the individual doctors. Nevertheless, the evidence suggested strongly that patients attending the nurse were much more likely to have had their educational needs met than if they only attended the doctor. It is assumed that this was because the nurse was more likely to follow the protocol than the doctors, she had longer appointments and she had received special instruction in demonstrating inhaler techniques.

Again we cannot be sure that every emergency nebulization was recorded, almost certainly some were not. But the figures were adequate to show that every patient at the practice in the sample requiring emergency treatment had either defaulted from treatment or had not yet been to the clinic; patients educated and established on treatment did not require such emergency care.

Managing change

The partners and nurse in the practice met to discuss the findings and agree an action plan (Table 11.7). They felt strongly that, on the evidence shown, asthma should be managed by the asthma nurse wherever possible. Their plan consisted of adding four items to the practice's asthma mangement plan, thus also adding four criteria on which care could be assessed.

Repeat

It was felt that probably the most important measure of success would be a reduction in hospital admissions and emergency treatment. All such episodes are currently being investigated to measure the number and whether some could have been avoided. The results are not yet available.

Table 11.7   *Plan following audit, 1990*

The asthma management protocol will be adapted by adding the following items:

1. The diagnosis should be entered into the computer in a standardized way to make retrieval easier.
2. All hospital admissions, emergency courses of oral steroids, and emergency nebulisations should also be entered in the records so that they can be studied.
3. The flow sheet must be used for everyone: it would be redesigned by the asthma nurse to make it easier to use.
4. All patients with asthma or suspected asthma should be referred to the nurse, including all hospital admissions following discharge.

ACKNOWLEDGEMENT

The data for the example of diabetic audit were kindly supplied by Dr Martin Lawrence.

REFERENCES

British Thoracic Society. (1990). Guidelines for management of asthma in adults. I Chronic persistent asthma. *British Medical Journal*, **301**, 651–3.

British Thoracic Society. (1990). Guidelines for management of asthma in adults. II Acute severe asthma. *British Medical Journal*, **301**, 797–800.

Cox, I. G. (1983). Treating diabetes and dementia. *British Medical Journal*, **287**, 1031–2.

Gellert, A. R., Gellert, S. L., and Illife, S. R. (1990). Prevalence and management of asthma in a London inner city general practice. *British Journal of General Practice*, **40**, 197–201.

Hayes, T. M. and Harries, J. (1984). Randomised controlled trial of routine hospital clinic care versus routine general practice care for type II diabetes. *British Medical Journal*, **289**, 728–30.

Levy, M. and Bell, L. (1984). General practice audit of asthma in childhood. *British Medical Journal*, **289**, 1115–16.

McKinnon, M. (1986). The role of nurses in general practice. *Practical Diabetes*, **3**, 232–4.

Singh, B. M. *et al.* (1984). Metabolic control of diabetes in general practice clinics: comparison with a hospital clinic. *British Medical Journal*, **289**, 726–8.

Speight, A. N. P., Lee, D. A., and Hey, E. N. (1983). Underdiagnosis and under-treatment of asthma in childhood. *British Medical Journal*, **286**, 1253–7.

12 Prescribing and formularies

Philip Reilly

There is no longer any doubt that audits of general practice prescribing in the UK will happen. The introduction of an indicative prescribing budget for each practice means that a crude form of external audit of prescribing is now in place. In such monitoring, cost is, of course, an immediate and important concern. The steeply rising expenditure on medications over recent years ensured that cost above all else would be considered in the health service reforms as they affect prescribing. UK prescribers are parsimonious in comparison to other similarly developed countries, but the large variation in the cost and frequency of prescribing by practices which were otherwise similar has interested the Government, which naturally sees the financial advantages of all practices behaving in the same way as the cheapest. The fact that such variations were and remain difficult to explain is only now being addressed.

Little in medical education prepares the doctor for prescribing in general practice. Young doctors have been thoroughly prepared theoretically and pharmacologically, but are unprepared either for the range of pathology or for some of the apparently irrational pressures to prescribe which occur in primary health care. Many older doctors fail to stay in touch with the rapidly changing field of modern therapeutics.

Competent prescribing implies:

(1) appropriate pharmacological and therapeutic knowledge;
(2) continuing access to relevant information about medications;
(3) communication skills with patients;
(4) the ability to maximize patient compliance;
(5) the ability to manage repeat prescribing systems.

Auditing with its essential strands of enumeration and evaluation has potential but largely undemonstrated educational impact. Currently the quantitative aspects of prescribing are very dominant. Cost containment with monthly budgetary statements feature very prominently in Government policy, and although lip service is paid to 'cost-effective' prescribing, there appears to be an assumption that the prescribing task is basically about reduction of prescribing frequency and above all about economy (Department of Health 1990). Little coherent response comes from the profession as a whole.

A small minority of doctors have consistently advocated a qualitative approach, with careful selection of medications. They have described the basis on which such a selection should be made in constructing formularies (Grant *et al.* 1985). Another school of thought, based outside the profession in the pharmaceutical industry, warns that patients may not be receiving the medications which they need (Teeling Smith 1991). It is a token of our predicament, when attempting to limit prescribing, that we have few answers to these arguments. The evaluative side of audit—the selecting of criteria for prescribing and the setting of the level of performance for compliance, so defining a standard—is so far poorly developed.

There are then two strategies which equip doctors to become competent prescribers and which also afford major opportunities of auditing prescribing: a quantitative approach through feedback of prescribing quantities and costs; and a qualitative approach through the development of formularies.

AUDIT OF PRESCRIBING: FEEDBACK SYSTEMS

Feedback systems are really massive data collecting systems for prescribing rates and costs. Prescribing Analysis and Cost (PACT) provides regular feedback on prescribing to general practitioners in England and Wales (Harris *et al.* 1990). The Scottish version (SPA) and the Northern Ireland version appeared on 1 April 1992.

PACT data is supplied at three levels of increasing complexity. PACT Level I sent to every practice each quarter. PACT Levels II and III are available on request (but PACT Level II is automatically sent to any practice with costs greater than 20 per cent above the local FHSA average). PACT Level I (Fig. 12.1) provides a practice with its overall prescribing costs in relation to the local FHSA average and the national average. It provides similar data for the six major therapeutic groups and it gives information on the proportion of medication prescribed generically. PACT Level II (Fig. 12.2) provides more detailed information showing the practice clearly in relationship to other local practices, and in addition, the amount and cost of prescribing for each drug category is provided. PACT Level III (Fig. 12.3) is a very detailed exposition of each doctor's prescribing behaviour giving the details of every item prescribed during one quarter tabulated under therapeutic categories.

Such feedback systems are passive, even when accompanied by comparative information. Moreover, there is no clinical or demographic data with which to interpret the crude prescribing data. To realize the potential of the system the data received must be evaluated in the context of the practice's social setting and clinical activity. Otherwise, the tendency will be for those with average prescribing to habituate, and those with costly prescribing to panic.

Choosing the topic

It is impossible to carry out detailed audit using all the PACT data. To make use of the data smaller areas have to be examined at any time, so that the whole of that clinical area can be reviewed. For example:

1. You and your colleagues notice that the practice is a very expensive prescriber of antihypertensives.

(a) Practice prescribing costs

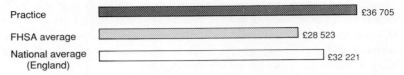

Practice	£36 705
FHSA average	£28 523
National average (England)	£32 221

Practice is above the FHSA average by £8182 or 29 per cent (and is above the national average by £4484 or 14 per cent).

(b) Percentage of items prescribed generically

Dr A	28%
Practice	26%
FHSA	44%
National	41%

(c) Practice items and total cost by major therapeutic group   Quarter ended Apr 1990

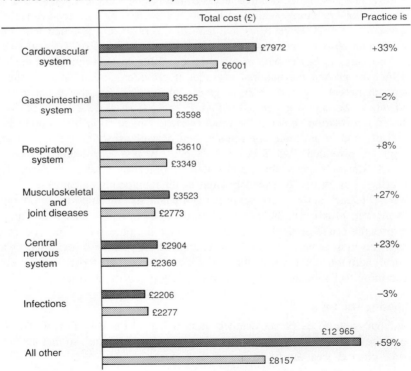

	Total cost (£)	Practice is
Cardiovascular system	£7972 / £6001	+33%
Gastrointestinal system	£3525 / £3598	−2%
Respiratory system	£3610 / £3349	+8%
Musculoskeletal and joint diseases	£3523 / £2773	+27%
Central nervous system	£2904 / £2369	+23%
Infections	£2206 / £2277	−3%
All other	£12 965 / £8157	+59%

Fig. 12.1   An example of the information provided by PACT Level I.

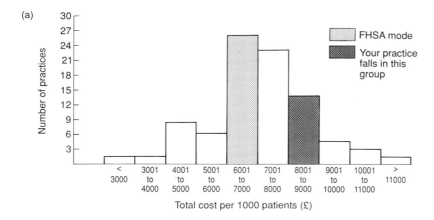

		Number of items	Cost (£)
	Total number of items and costs	521	3,610
3.1	Bronchodilators	326	1,754
3.2	Corticosteroids	113	1,501
3.3	Asthma prophylaxis	3	50
3.4	Allergic disorders	64	242
3.5	Respiratory stimulants	–	–
3.6	Oxygen	7	53
3.7	Mucolytics	–	–
3.8	Aromatic inhalations	–	–
3.9	Antitussives	5	5
3.10	Systematic nasal decongestants	3	7

Fig. 12.2 PACT Level II. (a) Distribution of practices in FHSA by total cost per 1000 patients. (b) Amount and prescribing cost for each drug category.

2. Your PACT data reveal that your practice is prescribing almost 50 per cent more items than the local average; however, the cost per item is barely three quarters of the local average.
3. Your costs in prescribing for the respiratory system are more than 40 per cent above the FHSA average. This may be related to an asthma clinic you run in the practice. It may be necessary to demonstrate that the clinic is cost-effective.

Collecting and evaluating the data

If the practice is concentrating on one specific area then it will be valuable to request PACT Level III information, so that practice's prescribing in that area can be reviewed in detail. To make sense of the prescribing data it must, however, be evaluated in conjunction with other practice information.

Hypnotics	Quantity	Number of prescriptions	Cost
Chlormethiazole			
Chlormethiazole edisylate	30	1	2.33
caps 192 mg	90	3	20.04
Heminevrin cap	100	2	14.84
Total		6	37.11
Nitrazepam			
Nitrazepam tab 5 mg	15	6	0.30
	20	3	0.21
	30	14	1.40
	40	15	2.10
	56	7	1.33
	60	24	4.80
Total		69	10.14
Temazepam			
Temazepam cap 10 mg	15	2	0.72
	20	2	0.96
	30	12	8.64
	40	6	5.76
	60	5	7.20
Temazepam cap 20 mg soft	28	4	4.72
Total		31	28.00
Triazolam			
Triazolam tab 125 μg	60	7	24.08
Total		7	24.08

Fig. 12.3   PACT Level III. Example: drugs prescribed by Dr A. in British National
Formulary category 4.1.1. (hypnotics).

1. Practice age profile.
   The precise age profile should be known, with as few 'ghost' patients as
   possible. Treatment of temporary residents should be noted if they are
   frequent. In respect of the elderly the weighting applied to PACT data (a
   factor of three for patients over 65 years) does not fully take account of
   increased costs of very elderly patients. Nursing homes could be a significant
   factor.
2. Local deprivation.
   Insofar as socio-economic deprivation is associated with increased morbidity
   and usage of medical care, then a knowledge of the practice making use of
   indices, such as the Jarman Index, is essential.
3. Morbidity.
   Chronic illness, especially respiratory, cardiovascular, and rheumatological,
   are all significant and should be quantified. Some conditions, such as cystic

fibrosis, AIDS, growth hormone deficiency, prostatic carcinoma, or intra-venous feeding, require expensive medications.
4. Interface with hospital.
   Various changes in secondary care delivery can affect general practice prescribing patterns. They include the discharge of certain vulnerable groups into the community; increasing day surgery; limited out-patient prescribing; hospital pharmacy policy, such as the prescribing of a drug available cheaply in hospital but expensively in the community.
5. Changes in clinical practice.
   Technological innovation can affect prescribing patterns, for instance erythropoetin or drugs for infertility treatment.
6. Repeat prescribing.
   At least one third of prescriptions are issued on a continuing basis, with the patient being seen only rarely. The elderly are the chief recipients of repeat prescriptions and the potential for side-effects, interactions, and non-compliance are considerable.
7. Areas of special interest.
   A practice may have an active screening programme for hypertension or hyperlipidaemia, or may be especially interested in managing particular groups of patients, for instance asthmatics. The cost of medication for patients can be high, but there is evidence of benefit, and a vigorous proactive approach should be encouraged. The high cost of such care places increased onus on doctors to audit their performance with both process measurements (for example, coverage for follow-up) and outcomes (for example, peak flow readings and admission rates).

In the light of this type of practice information the PACT data and the topics selected can be better evaluated.

For example, *topic*: the practice is a high prescriber of antihypertensives.

Evaluation: the practice has a hypertension clinic. In view of the expensive costs this clinic needs to be reviewed. How does our detection rate compare with published figures in other practices? Are patients fully evaluated prior to being started on treatment? Are there arrangements for review and considering drug withdrawal if the blood pressure falls? Is there a practice policy on first line, second line drugs, and on referral? Is all medication being given generically? Are the hospitals beginning medication which the practice does not wish to use?

Topic: the practice is prescribing 50 per cent more items, but cheaper, than the local average.

Evaluation: does the practice have an abnormally high consultation rate? What are patients' expectations? Are there cultural or ethnic reasons? Do the doctors have recognized reasons for prescribing? Is there a practice policy for managing self-limiting illness?

Topic: the practice runs an asthma clinic and has respiratory system prescribing costs 40 per cent above the FHSA average.

Evaluation: what proportion of patients are recorded as asthmatic? Is there evidence of compliance with review appointments? Is there evidence that the asthma control has benefited from increased medication? Does the practice protocol use the most cost-effective preparations?

Planning care and implementing change

In the light of this evaluation the practice members may decide on a policy of care for the topic being considered, and this may involve some changes. There is no doubt that a plan of care needs to be written if adherence is to be achieved, and any plan for altering prescribing is unlikely to be successfully implemented unless it is part of a plan for the overall management of the topic under consideration.

When practices are observed examining their own prescribing data they progress or fail to progress through a series of stages (Reilly 1985).

1. Defensive comments: for example, 'We are not very good at this'.
2. Projective comments: for example, 'We are the sort of practice which . . .'.
3. Deficiency acknowledged: this is especially seen when the group has its own data available.
4. Dialogue.
5. Agreement/diasagreement: this depends on openness, and the ability to give and receive criticism.
6. Policy development: the practice group needs some form of working consensus as well as good sources of information.
7. Implementation of change.
   Check that change has taken place: repeat of the audit.

Practice groups will not progress beyond the stage of agreement/disagreement unless they work together regularly and in a manner which caters for the needs of the team members as well as the task in hand.

The management of change and the development of innovation are demanding. The practice needs to know why change is really necessary. The whole process must seem and actually be possible. The impression and the reality will be more successful if the whole process is shared by all the participants. Both practice and individual partner identity will be reinforced.

Agreeing criteria and repeating the cycle

It is difficult to agree criteria and levels of performance for a topic as difficult to assess as personal prescribing, but certain crude criteria may be set. For instance, it may be agreed to introduce more generic prescribing: to set a definite policy on first and second line antihypertensives medications: or to attempt to reduce prescribing for self-limiting illness. PACT Level I will provide information on the proportion of prescribing which is generic: PACT Level II will give some indication of success in attaining targets for such matters as reducing overall prescribing: for an indication of success in meeting more detailed guidelines, such as adhering to practice policy for antihypertensives, the practice will have to request PACT Level III.

AUDIT OF PRESCRIBING: FORMULARIES

Choosing the topic

A second strategy which equips doctors to become competent prescribers and also affords major opportunities for audit of prescribing is that of formulary construction. Formularies are voluntary preferred selections of medications made by the prescribers (McGavock *et al.* 1988). Such a strategy involves active involvement in developing a prescribing policy (Reilly *et al.* 1989).

General practitioners largely manage common illnesses, and a large majority of these will respond to an established medication. Most patients receiving established medications are treated cost-effectively without in any way receiving second rate medications. In managing the minority of patients not responding to established medications, the prescriber can be appropriately radical, outside the formulary selection—formularies in general practice must imply flexibility. Such a professional approach from the prescriber means that patients get the medications appropriate to their clinical condition.

Planning care

It is relatively easy to list the characteristics a drug must possess. Effective, safe, economic, appropriate to the patient's condition, acceptable, and free of side-effects. It is, however, quite a challenge to use these items in making a choice between the various preparations in a given therapeutic class.

One approach is to list specific selection criteria for the various drugs under consideration. (Table 12.1) (Herxheimer 1976).

The names of the medications being reviewed are placed across the top of the sheet. For each one its characteristics in relation to the listed criteria are stated. The group selecting the drugs for the formulary—which may benefit from including a pharmacist—can quickly see the profiles of the drugs. The drugs having the most acceptable profiles are then selected.

In constructing formularies certain principles have been evolved (Grant *et al.* 1985). They include:

1. Adequate treatment must be available for the majority of patients.
2. The formulary must be acceptable to the general practitioners using it.
3. Generic prescribing should be encouraged.
4. New medicines should be avoided until firm evidence is available for advantages over existing medicines.

Table 12.1 *Selection criteria for drugs under consideration*

	Names of various medications			
	Drug A	Drug B	Drug C	etc.
Aim (in use)				
Observations				
Alternatives				
Duration of course				
Metabolism				
Interactions				
Route and dosage				
Unwanted effects				
Cost				

5. Cost. This is important but has to be assessed in relation to benefit.
6. Regular updating must be planned.

Practices may find it helpful to consult some of the formularies already developed as a starting point for developing their own (Lothian Liaison Committee 1989).

Many prescribing issues will be raised and not all can be settled. The selection process must be ongoing and is a major learning opportunity in which doctors use a structured approach for selection both of established and new medications.

Setting target standards

Constructing a formulary is an educational exercise; determining adherence to that formulary is an exercise in audit. The practice is likely to set a criterion that in each prescribing class the drugs prescribed should come from the practice formulary. As suggested above the target level of performance for adhering to that formulary should be at least 80 per cent. Some of the items vary hugely in cost and a practice may aim for greater adherence in the more expensive drug classes.

Observe practice and analyse data

There are three main ways of collecting data to test adherence to a formulary. *Either* PACT Level III can be requested, and the practice usage for a particular therapeutic use assessed; *or* a practice computer can be searched for recent prescribing behaviour so long as all medication is recorded *or* the doctors can keep records of prescriptions, or duplicate prescriptions, and then analyse them.

One practitioner or member of staff is likely to have the responsibility for collecting the information for feedback to a whole group of doctors at a practice

Example 1 145

meeting. Although all the practice may be involved in receiving requests for, recommending, or dispensing medicines, only the doctors can prescribe. So it may be that the appropriate group for analysing this audit is that of the doctors alone — especially if threatening personal comparisons are being made.

Implement change and repeat the cycle

It may be that the practice achieves its target for keeping to the formulary: it may fail. Alternatively, some doctors may have success and other fail. Various options are then open. If the variation of performance between doctors is great, then discussion may enable some doctors to change their behaviour to that of more successful doctors; alternatively, if the target is achieved very easily, then this may be because the formulary is too lax; or maybe the target has not been achieved, not because of the poor behaviour of the doctors, but because the formulary is too restrictive and needs broadening in order to provide a reasonable range of options.

EXAMPLE 1

A four doctor training practice developed a formulary and decided to audit adherence to the formulary. It was agreed to do the assessment in March, as all the doctors were usually present then and the workload was steady. The method used was to produce duplicate prescriptions; either by using carbon paper in surgery or on visits, or by producing duplicates on the practice computer which is used for repeat prescriptions. The doctors also recorded consultations ending with no prescription. The prescripions were examined by a staff member who recorded both the total number of items, and then the number which were for drugs not included in the formulary.

Data collection

After the first (1989) data collection a practice meeting met to examine:

(1) the variation between doctors;
(2) the frequency with which consultations ended without prescription;
(3) drugs to be removed from the formulary;
(4) drugs to be added to the formulary.

Following the second (1991) collection it was clear that:

(1) the number of consultations ending with no prescription had risen;
(2) the compliance with the formulary was over 90 per cent for all partners.

The results are shown in Table 12.2.

Table 12.2   *Results of data collection in 1989 and 1991*

	Dr L/Dr N		Dr D		Dr J		Dr R		Trainee	
	1989	1991	1989	1991	1989	1991	1989	1991	1989	1991
Number of patients seen	338	485	472	434	486	490	249	298	172	330
Number with no prescription	94	155	172	188	188	127	58	90	92	122
Number of items conforming	260	254	322	301	307	435	230	250	93	228
Percentage given no prescription	28	53	36	43	39	26	23	30	53	37
Percentage conforming	85	95	77	94	89	94	91	94	92	87

There will always be a relationship between the size of the formulary and the degree of conformity. Since the practice has low costs in relation to local practices it is unlikely that the formulary is too generous. The practice intends to continue its practice policy and review again in two years. (Dr A. Dunnill and Partners, East Oxford Health Centre.)

EXAMPLE 2

Topic: a nine doctor practice co-operated with three local chemists to audit the effect of introducing a formulary.

Data collection: the chemists checked all antibiotic prescriptions for one month (February 1986). It was estimated that this would be at least 85 per cent of the practice's total.

Data evaluated and care planned: a formulary was developed using the expertise of two partners, the local hospital pharmacist, a literature search, and the evidence of current usage. It was submitted to the other members of the partnership and the local pharmacists for comment and agreement.

Data collection: after one year the data collection exercise was repeated (Table 12.3).

Evaluation

1. In 1986 the top six antibiotics accounted for 79 per cent of the total, in 1987 for 89 per cent.
2. Co-trimoxazole fell from second to seventh, trimethoprim rose from fourteenth to second.

Table 12.3 *Results of data collection after one year*

	Number of items		Cost	
	February 1986	February 1987	February 1986	February 1987
*Amoxycillin	168	194	585	510
Co-trimoxazole	73	10	231	19
*Penicillin V	57	69	23	25
*Erythromycin	50	81	115	215
*Flucloxacillin	48	35	270	223
*Oxytetracycline	31	26	15	17
Cephalosporins	20	3	90	26
Amoxycillin/ clavanulate	4	0	35	0
*Trimethoprim	4	93	1	31
Total	537	559	1769	1334

*Drugs included in the practice formulary.

3. The use of certain antibiotics not in the formulary fell to zero.
4. Cost saving in one month was £435, or 25 per cent.

Plan of care

It was agreed that the formulary had produced more unified care and considerable cost savings without any apparent detriment to the patients. It was agreed to continue the policy, but in view of the strong compliance it was agreed that the formulary should be regularly reviewed to ensure that new drugs whose efficacy became demonstrated would be included as appropriate (Needham *et al.* 1988).

REFERENCES

Department of Health (England and Wales). (1990). *Improving prescribing 1990.* Department of Health, London.
Grant, G. B., Gregory, D. A., and van Zwanenberg, T. D. (1985). Development of a limited formulary for general practice. *Lancet*, **1**, 1030–2.
Harris, C. M., Heywood, P. L., and Clayden, A. D. (1990). *The analysis of prescribing in general practice. A guide to audit and research.* HMSO, London.
Herxheimer, A. (1976). Towards parity for therapeutics in clinical teaching. Questions to ask yourself about drugs. *Lancet*, **ii**, 1186.

Lothian Liaison Committee Prescribing Group. (1989). *Lothian Formulary No. 2.* Ladywell Medical Centre, Edinburgh.

McGavock, H., Woods, J., Reilly, P. M. *et al.* (1988). *Practice formulary 1988–1990.* N. Ireland Faculty RCGP.

Reilly, P. M. (1985). An audit of prescribing by peer review. Unpublished M.D. thesis: Queen's University, Belfast.

Reilly, P. M., Gilleghan, J. D., Horner, R., and Eckersley, A. P. R. (1989). *How to produce a practice formulary.* RCGP, London.

Needham, A., Brown, M., and Freeborn, S. (1988). Introduction and audit of a general practice antibiotic formulary. *Journal of the Royal College of General Practice*, **38**, 166–7.

Teeling-Smith, G. (1991). *Patterns of prescribing.* Office of Health Economics, London.

13 Critical incident analysis: cases and patterns

Thomas O'Dowd

In the first chapter of his book *Epidemiology in country practice*, William Pickles grabs attention with the following account:

A gypsy woman driving a caravan into a village in the summer twilight, a sick husband in the caravan, a faulty pump at which she proceeded to wash her dirty linen, and my first and only serious epidemic of typhoid left me with a lasting impression of the unique opportunities of the country doctor for the investigation of infectious disease. (Pickles 1983)

Pickles was aware of the importance of examining a critical and unusual event in his practice. Because of his knowledge of the Broad Street pump he was able to interpret and understand that event, and use it to make a change which would improve the health of his patients in Wensleydale.

The single interesting case in medicine has a long tradition, from historical descriptions of disease to the present day grand round in the teaching hospital. Doctors and medical students are more strongly influenced by anecdotes than by the denominator from which we choose them. Experienced clinical teachers will bring a subject to life for undergraduate medical students by citing a recent interesting case, noting points of agreement with, and deviation from, the textbooks. Case reporting is a sizeable section of many specialist journals; for example, the widely respected *New England Journal of Medicine* runs a weekly clinico-pathological conference on an interesting case that ends up in the post-mortem room.

In primary care much of the importance of the critical incident is that it has gone against expectations: it disturbs the calm expectation of the practice that everything is under control. For this reason, analysis of a single critical event may demonstrate more scope for improvement than many routine surveys involving large numbers.

RANDOM CASE ANALYSIS

In his pioneering work with general practitioners, Michael Balint used a case-based approach which concentrated on the triad of doctor, patient, and illness. (Balint 1957) This approach emphasized the individuality of each clinical transaction. This has had benefits and disadvantages in the use of cases to develop doctors' education and patients' care.

Balint's influence has given general practitioners a sophistication in case analysis, particularly evident in the widespread and effective use of random case discussion as a teaching tool between the trainer and the trainee. Buckley (1990) has described that, at its simplest, random case analysis merely requires a list of patients seen at the end of a recent surgery session which are then discussed. Buckley has listed five questions that can be almost universally used in random case analysis.

1. Has the clinical problem been clearly identified?
2. Have underlying or continuing problems been declared or explored?
3. What are the expectations of the patient from the consultation?
4. Do we have adequate information about the clinical problem?
5. How does the doctor feel about the consultation?

Conversely, the emphasis accorded by Balint to the potential of every consultation for analysis and to the individuality of each case has given the impression that any case is a good as another for discussion. This has perhaps distracted practitioners from the need to concentrate on particularly critical incidents, and from the potential of aggregating cases to find a common pattern.

CRITICAL INCIDENTS

Reviewing critical or significant incidents in general practice is increasingly being used as a method of audit. Daily practice life is full of events that are unexpected, disturbing, funny, and sad. When do such events become significant? Is the review of such an event audit anyway? A critical incident is one that affects the practice over and above the routine, that has the potential to be examined, learned from, and which will perhaps alter the ways of doing things in future. By examining such an event we can reveal an aspect of our practice which is in need of change. Significant events are likely to lead the practice into self education and research as they reveal lack of knowledge in the practice or information in the literature. There may be few other standards to compare with, and the practice may have to develop standards in a particular area that may be useful to others.

A critical event may be clinical or non-clinical and may affect any member of the practice. There are traditional topics, such as cardiovascular accidents or myocardial infarctions, which may have been preventable. The idea is that the members of the practice will meet to discuss such cases while they are fresh in their memory backed up by the case notes. Questions such as 'How preventable was it?', 'How did the practice deal with the clinical event and the family?' can be addressed, and any deficiencies noted and practice policy changed as a result.

There are, however, events other than clinical events that are important to a practice. Do patients who change practice but not address tell us anything about our practice? If we are the recipient of such patients do we wish to encourage this and what is our attraction? To measure this may mean gathering information at a new patient interview for discussion later to compare with the experience of others in the practice. If we are the losers of such patients it is equally important to reflect, and discussion with clinical and non-clinical staff may reveal a reason that explains the loss. Needless to say, only the most robust of groups may feel they are able to carry out this type of case audit, as difficulties such as availability, access, clinical performance, and staff training may emerge.

Night work will probably be a popular item of audit because of the steep rise of such demand in many practices. A general audit of night visits may only reveal that they are increasing: for a real understanding of what is going on, specific events or groups of calls may have to be examined. For instance, it may be found that certain types of families generate calls. If families new to the area generate many calls the practice may wish to examine its introductory leaflet and perhaps its support through the nurses or health visitors. Acting on information learned in auditing critical incidents in this way may well be beneficial to the quality of life of the partners.

Some patients complain that doctors do not listen to them. This is a frequent complaint that leaves doctors floundering, especially when they are putting effort and training into good communication. What are the characteristics of patients who say their doctors don't listen, and what do they really want? An audit of a few cases may reveal that patients have had an adequate amount of physical examination and laboratory testing, but that they are left with the idea that their story does not matter (Charlton 1991). Such patients are unlikely to complain directly to the doctor they feel is not listening, but instead to a partner or a hospital colleague. To do an audit of this kind would mean having to be open enough to identify both patients and doctors. The patients may well be right, and an individual doctor has indeed stopped listening, which is why such audit is so threatening but potentially useful.

Analysis of significant events can enter the audit cycle just like other areas of medical audit. It requires an event to be observed or remarked upon in the practice. Discussion may be diffuse initially, but with effective chairmanship or leadership the significant items may be distilled into areas that can be measured. If at this stage the prime mover in the group briefly records what was discussed and extracts the areas of interest on to a flowsheet for action the practice is on the first rung of an interesting audit. The practice should make plans for ways in which similar events will be handled in the future, and even if an identical case does not occur again, certain general principles may be decided. Of course, repeating the cycle cannot apply to an individual event, but once one case has been reviewed, similar ones often arise.

CRITICAL EVENTS: AN EXAMPLE

During surgery hours a member of staff is detailed to handle prescription queries, liaise with hospitals, and take requests for visits. Practice policy was that reception staff were not required to request clinical details, although most patients offer some details. If the patient stated that he or she needed urgent help then the request was passed to doctor on call for that day and responded to appropriately.

Mrs Emily Johnson is a 59-year-old widow living alone in a downstairs flat in a small housing estate. Just after nine o'clock on a Monday morning she telephoned and requested if the doctor could 'pop in and see me', her full address was taken and her medical file was placed along with the other requests for visits.

Mrs Johnson was visited just after two o'clock that afternoon and was found to be having severe chest pain of 7–8 hour duration, shocked, and in need of urgent hospital admission. She survived a large myocardial infarction and on being visited on return to her home was extremely grateful to her doctor for sending her into hospital.

The event was discussed in detail because it had revealed a serious organizational flaw that almost led to a calamity for Mrs Johnson. The event had a 'there but for the grace of God go I' effect on the partners and led to an immediate change in the way requests for visits are handled. The partners still felt strongly about reception staff not requesting clinical details, but they agreed to speak to all patients requesting a visit, giving advice and an approximate time of visiting. It does entail yet another intrusion into consulting time, but has also meant a small decrease in home visits, as some patients find that they can make it to surgery following discussion on the telephone with the doctor.

Of course the partners could have adopted the course of allowing the receptionist more freedom in eliciting clinical details from patients requesting home visits. This would have opened up the area of staff responsibility and training. In the event the partners reacted by taking the responsibility on themselves, which is all too often a professional response.

Mrs Johnson's critical incident elicited a response from the partners which developed practice policy. It also revealed a reactive way of dealing with the incident which was both hierarchical and authoritarian. The further significance of this event was that it revealed a management style that perhaps needs examination and re-evaluation.

DEVELOPING PATTERNS

Critical incident discussion is an evocative and powerful way of looking at what Marinker (1987) calls 'the interior of general practice'. We naturally wish to discuss such incidents because they trouble, exasperate, or frustrate us. But the greatest value of such cases is when they begin to fit together, to produce a pattern from which we can make resolutions and plans for practice which alter the future management of similar situations for the better.

We are inexperienced in finding a theme for the cases that we discuss with colleagues. Finding a pattern in cardiology for instance, is relatively easy: there is an international measure of consensus about diagnoses and management allowing standards to be set and measured. This consensus allows cardiologists in Berlin the scope to discuss cases, advances, and ideas with colleagues in London or Tokyo. It allows specialists to think in explicit terms and provides a forum for integrating cases into wider experience. In general practice we pride ourselves in operating in grey, uncertain areas. We use these areas as our charisma to demonstrate the interesting nature of our work. However, we are in danger of making part of our work inaccessible and mysterious when it should be neither.

In general practice we are short of the skills necessary to identify patterns in the varied and interesting diversity of our work. Until we encourage the development of such skills and ways of thinking there are boundaries to improvement in our care which need not be there. Can the cases we discuss be linked together into a series? Can our cases become accessible to standard setting? Instead of our free-standing cases can we develop a method to link horizontally the cases that puzzle or defy our clinical expertise? Instead of Mrs Jones with the bad back, can we reframe the problem into 'backs that won't get better'. Instead of Mr Smith who always wants referral, is it possible to measure the number of patient initiated referrals in the practice and then deal with any questions arising from such a measurement.

This can be a natural progression from critical incident analysis. The observation of one critical incident may reverberate in the experience of members of the care team, and by exciting their interest and imagination may encourage them to report similar cases so that a pattern may develop.

AN EXAMPLE—THE HEARTSINK AUDIT

Every general practitioner has patients on his or her list who cause exasperation and that familiar feeling of being overwhelmed when their names are seen on the appointments book. Such patients have become known as heartsink patients (O'Dowd 1988) and the term has rapidly entered the medical lexicon despite slightly pejorative overtones. Doctors experience anticipatory anxiety before such patients consult (McDonald and O'Dowd 1991), and they are, by and large, a desperate group of people whose only common denominator is the emotional reaction they provoke in the doctor. The term 'heartsink' was one that was used frequently by general practitioners in a Welsh practice and it gave rise to a useful theme on which to base a study of difficult patients.

A group of 28 patients who were causing particular stress to a practice in South Wales were identified. They seemed dissatisfied with the services provided, placed many demands on the practice and were frequent attenders with seemingly endless complaints. Data was collected to summarize their reasons for attending. Present management was outlined if apparent and the findings were presented at team meetings. At each meeting partners shared information and defined apparent problems. A management plan was evolved which was recorded in the patient's notes and subsequent meetings were held to review progress. The management plan arose from shared knowledge and was tailored for each patient. The main targets were to assess the size of the problem and to make the patients less heartsink by gaining an understanding of them. There were spin-offs—the numbers were much smaller than feared—consultation rates declined, and on review five years later the managed group were considered much less heartsink by the practice. The interest and expertise built up has been of considerable benefit to the doctors' practice and the management of such patients has been shared with the profession.

The heartsink story is an example of one significant case being joined to others to make a series. The series arose because of distress caused to the practice by difficult patients. Such an area has been capable of entering the audit cycle, plans were made for management, and targets were set. Five years later another measurement took place and it was possible to audit how the partners then felt about the same heartsink patients. The medical profession is accustomed to outcome measures of a scientific nature. Professional feelings as an outcome measure are usually confined to psychotherapy, but when used in our discipline may be every bit as helpful and as diagnostic as a blood result or fibreoptic finding.

CONCLUSION

It will be a pity if audit is used as a narrow method of measuring those things about general practice that occur frequently and are easy to measure. It is a mistake to say that much of what we do cannot be measured. We spend much time telling each other about critical cases and incidents but when it comes to audit we often try to measure the commonplace. Auditing critical incidents and developing patterns from such cases will help every practice team to define and improve its care.

REFERENCES

Balint, M. (1957). *The doctor, his patient, and the illness*. Pitman, London.
Buckley, G. (1990). Clinically significant events. *In Medical audit and general practice*, (ed. M. Marinker), pp. 121–7, British Medical Journal, London.
Charlton, B. G. (1991). Stories of sickness. *British Journal of General Practice*, **41**, 222–3.
Marinker, M. (1987). Journey to the interior: the search for academic general practice. *Journal of the Royal College of General Practitioners*, **37**, 385–7.
McDonald, P. S. and O'Dowd, T. C. (1991). The heartsink patient: a preliminary study. *Family Practice*, **8**(2), 112–16.
O'Dowd, T. C. (1988). Five years of heartsink patients in general practice. *British Medical Journal*, **297**, 528–30.
Pickles, W. N. (1984). Epidemiology in country practice. *Royal College of General Practitioners*, London.

14 Problem-solving audits

Martin Lawrence

'Problems', writes Baker (1990), 'can be thought of as deficiencies that those in the practice think are so important that corrective action must be taken'. He goes on to express the view that audits done in response to acknowledged problems usually result in change, those done for curiosity or under compulsion are less likely to do so. Since the prime aim of audit is to improve care, this implies that problem-solving audits are likely to be the most fruitful.

Significant event analysis and problem solving have a great deal in common. The former can be construed as formal review of a specific incident, seeking changes which might enable a similar situation to be handled better in future; the latter as an investigation set up to analyse a problem—which may indeed have been revealed by an event.

Not only are problem-solving audits likely to produce change, they can often be small and manageable. This is a great encouragement for practices beginning to do audit: the data may be collected and analysed in a short time while the interest is still alive; changes resulting from the evaluation can be introduced soon after the topic was proposed, so that team members see the relevance; and the work may be light enough and straightforward enough for any member of the team to carry out, perhaps the person who reported the problem.

This chapter offers a few very simple audits as examples. In each case a practice has identified a problem and used audit as a means of defining the problem so as to implement rational change. Indeed the initials of problem-solving audit (PSA) are the same as for perfectly simple audit, which is the subject of the first example.

EXAMPLE 1 CONTACT WITH THE ELDERLY

Problem

On a day of severe snow a general practitioner became concerned as to how many elderly patients (over 80 years of age) could be contacted by telephone to check whether they were coping.

Data collection

A review of the medical records showed that only 15 per cent had a telephone number recorded.

Plan

It was decided to search the telephone book and use directory enquiries to improve the rate of recording.

Target standard

A recording level of at least 80 per cent was set, leaving few to be contacted in other ways.

Second data collection

By midday, telephone numbers were available in 85 per cent of the records of patients aged over 80 years.

Plan

Volunteers were sent round to visit the 15 per cent of patients who could not be contacted by telephone.

Conclusion

A very simple audit exercise, which took less than a day, resulted in the practice being able to contact every patient aged over 80 years in adverse weather conditions. The audit is simple to repeat in order to ensure that the service is maintained.

Dr Smith, in the *Journal of the Royal College*, emphasizes that PSAs (perfectly simple audits) can be as useful as FCAs (frightfully clever audits).

(Dr Colin Smith, Marshlands Practice, Higham, Kent, UK)

EXAMPLE 2   TERMINATION OF PREGNANCY

Problem

A practice became concerned about the care given to patients having termination of pregnancy.

1. Was contraceptive care adequate, before and after termination of pregnancy?
2. Was management of anti-D administration foolproof?
3. Could the audit be used to check the practice's rubella programme?

Targets

1. All patients should have had contraceptive advice.
2. All patients should have received contraceptive advice after termination of pregnancy.

Example 2 Termination of pregnancy 157

3. All patients should have their blood group recorded as part of the procedure.
4. All Rhesus negative patients should have had anti-D following termination of pregnancy.
5. The rubella status of all patients of child-bearing age should be recorded in their notes.

Data collection

A total of 29 patients had 30 terminations of pregnancy in the year prior to audit day. Data for these patients were as follows:

1. Consultation in previous year: nil = 6, once = 1, twice or more = 23.
2. Contraceptive advice in previous year: nil = 20, once = 5, twice or more = 5.
3. Contraceptive advice after termination of pregnancy: nil = 6, once = 12, twice or more = 12.
4. Blood group known following termination of pregnancy: no = 7, yes = 23.
5. Anti-D administration known: no = 20, yes = 10.
6. Rubella status known: no = 5, yes = 25.

Evaluation and plan

1. Knowledge of rubella status is good, but three 'unknowns' had consulted in the previous year. *Plan*: Rubella immunity should be checked routinely at consultations.
2. A total of 80 per cent of patients returned for contraceptive advice, but not all did so. *Plan*: All women should be invited for contraceptive advice after termination of pregnancy.
3. The best information of blood group and anti-D administration came from the Pregnancy Advisory Service. *Plan*: Establish procedure with NHS and private gynaecologists for blood group and anti-D administration to be included in the discharge letter.

Targets

1. Information on blood group and anti-D administration should be in all discharge letters.
2. Rubella status information should be recorded for all women of child-bearing age.
3. All women should attend for contraceptive advice after termination of pregnancy.

(Dr J. C. Hasler, Sonning Common Health Centre, Berks, UK)

EXAMPLE 3   ANTIBIOTIC TREATMENT OF RESPIRATORY TRACT INFECTION

Problem

A seven doctor practice with personal lists became concerned about excessive and varied prescribing for respiratory tract infection.

Data collection

It was agreed to collect data on prescribing for respiratory tract infections, excluding sinusitis, until 50 cases had been seen by each doctor. The following pattern was found:

Prescription	Doctor						
	A	B	C	D	E	F	G
Penicillin V	7	11	9	13	8	20	13
Amoxycillin	16	18	17	19	5	17	15
Erythromycin	5	6	3	4	1	2	0
Tetracyclines	9	5	8	0	1	2	5
Other	3	1	1	3	3	2	5
No prescription	10	9	12	11	32	7	12

Evaluation

The data was discussed at a partners' clinical meeting.

1. It was noted that the pattern of prescribing was similar, although older doctors used more tetracyclines, and younger doctors more penicillin.
2. It was noted that one doctor was particularly successful at not prescribing. He was especially keen on patient education.
3. Branded amoxycillin, erthromycin, and tetracyclines were used by some doctors. It was agreed to prefer penicillin V, amoxycillin, oxytetracycline, and trimethoprim.

Plan

The partners agreed to concentrate their effort on the management of sore throats. Dr E would draw up a practice protocol to emphasize patient education. A practice leaflet would be produced (Fig. 14.1).

Advice on dealing with sore throats

The vast majority of sore throats will get better without any treatment that needs a doctor's prescription. More sore throats are due to viruses, which are not killed by antibiotics (such as penicillin) but are destroyed in time by the body's natural defence mechanisms. Simple measures will usually keep a sore throat sufferer fairly comfortable while nature does the rest.

This advice leaflet is *not* intended as a substitute for a medical consultation–if the patient (or parents) are unsure of the seriousness of the illness.

Symptoms

Sore throats may or may not be part of a 'cold', and may be accompanied by any of the following:

(1) temperature (fever)
(2) headache
(3) aches and pains in the limbs
(4) runny nose
(5) cough
(6) sickness and diarrhoea (or mild 'upset stomach', especially in children).

Most sore throats and accompanying symptoms will be much improved in about 5 days, but an irritating cough may easily persist for 2–3 weeks. Smoking in the household is likely to worsen this symptom.

Treatment

Rest is an important part of the treatment. Children who are unwell should not be sent to school.

Plenty to drink, for example diluted fruit juice, barley water, etc., especially if there is a temperature, diarrhoea, or sickness.

Do not force food –the appetite will soon return, once the patient feels better.

Warm drinks, throat pastilles, and throat sprays all are soothing.

Fever control is important, particularly in the *under 5s*, some of whom may be liable to convulsions when feverish for any reason. In case of febrile convulsion, place the child on its side at once and seek advice.

Ways of bringing down temperature (fever control)

1. Removal of most *or* all clothing and bedding *plus* good ventilation–open windows, use a fan or blow heater, or hair dryer on *cold.*

2. *Tepid sponging* –remove all the child's clothing, sit or stand the child in bath or bowl of lukewarm water and spong water over the whole body repeatedly, allowing water to evaporate from the surface of the body. This is the quickest method of cooling a very feverish patient. It should be effective in 15–20 minutes.

3. *Medicines* are useful but can take up to an hour to act, so use *tepid sponging as well* if there is an urgent need to reduce the temperature.

For babies over 3 months and children under 12 years
Do give paracetamol elixir (Calpol, Disprol) for relief of pain and temperature. Repeat every four hours as necessary. *Do not give aspirin in any form.*

For feverish babies under 3 months:
Must *not* be given paracetamol elixir (calpol, Disprol) *or* aspirin. Keep clothing and coverings to a minimum, and use tepid sponging if necessary.

Adults

Two soluble aspirins dissolved in water is an effective remedy, and can be repeated every four hours as necessary. Some people use it as a gargle before swallowing.
Two soluble paracetamol for adults who cannot take aspirin, (for example asthmatics, stomach ulcer sufferers, and people *allergic* to aspirin), may be taken in a similar way.

Note: antibiotics
Recent scientific research has shown that antibiotics are of much less value in the treatment of sore throats than previously thought, and the doctors in the Windrush Health Centre are trying to reduce unnecessary prescribing of these drugs.

Fig. 14.1 An example of a patient information leaflet.

Target

1. The number of patients receiving no treatment for respiratory tract infection should be higher, at least 50 per cent.
2. Penicillin, amoxycillin, oxytetracycline, and trimethoprim should be the drugs of choice (the practice did not set a target level).

Data collection

The data collection exercise was repeated 12 months later. On this occasion, the data were collected for two weeks instead of until 50 cases had been seen. This revealed marked variations in the numbers of patients seen (8–39), as shown below:

Prescription	Doctor					
	A	B	C	D	E	F*
Penicillin V	8	5	1	6	2	0
Amoxycillin	4	1	0	7	1	7
Erythromycin	3	0	0	6	0	0
Tetracyclines	1	0	2	0	0	1
Other	1	0	2	0	0	0
No prescription	14	8	9	10	22	0

The percentage of patients who received no treatment in the two surveys was compared, as shown below:

	Percentage of patients receiving no treatment					
Doctor	A	B	C	D	E	F*
Survey 1	20	18	24	22	64	14
Survey 2	46	57	64	34	88	0

*Dr F had changed from a retired to a new partner between surveys.

Evaluation

1. A higher proportion of penicillin V was prescribed, but amoxycillin remained popular (expecially with the new Dr F).
2. The large variation in the number of patients seen could be due to expectation of response, but may also be due to different labelling of patients' conditions by the doctors.

Example 4   Control of patients taking warfarin   161

3. It is intriguing that the doctor who prescribed least was consulted for the condition most.
4. Clearly, the proportion of patients not receiving a prescription rose between the audit.

Plan

1. The previously planned policy to be continued.
2. The new partner must be introduced to the practice policy.
3. The review to be repeated again in two years.

Conclusion

The methodology has not been validated, but the figures are sufficient to encourage the doctors that their first audit has produced change, and to encourage them to further effort.

(Dr P. G. Kay and partners, Windrush Surgery, Witney, Oxon, UK)

EXAMPLE 4   CONTROL OF PATIENTS TAKING WARFARIN

Problem

Two patients had suffered major problems following drug interactions with warfarin. The practice decided to review warfarin management, especially with regard to:

(1) reasons for the use of warfarin;
(2) frequency of complications;
(3) completeness of follow-up.

Data collection

A total of 47 patients were on warfarin, as shown below:

Reason for use		Duration of use	
Deep vein thrombosis (DVT) and		<2 years	21
pulmonary embolism	16	2–10 years	16
Atrial fibrillation	12	>10 years	9
Valvular disease	10		
Dyskinetic left ventricle	3		
Other	5		

45 patients had had prothrombin checked within one month.
17 patients had 50 per cent of prothrombin results outside the guideline range.
3 patients had suffered drug interactions (2 asapropazone, 1 phenylbutazone).
Several patients were on polypharmacy (amiodarone, aspirin, phenytoin).
There was no serious bleeding.

Evaluation

The overall quality of follow-up was good. The main problems were of control
due to:

(1) individual patient variation;
(2) known or unexpected drug interactions.

Changes introduced

1. Each patient to have a prothrombin chart with the target therapeutic range
    highlighted at the top (2—2.5 for prophylaxis of DVT; 2—3 for treatment of
    DVT, pulmonary embolism, atrial fibrillation; 3—4.5 for recurrent DVT,
    pulmonary embolism, valves or grafts).
2. All medications to be listed at the top of the prothrombin chart.
3. Blood for prothrombin tests to be taken on days when the patient's own
    doctor is available in the evening to manage control.
4. Patients to telephone on the evening of a prothrombin test for follow-up
    instructions.
5. 'Patient on warfarin' to be highlighted in the patient's notes.

Conclusion

This audit was reassuring inasmuch at it showed good follow-up of patients on
warfarin, but concerning because despite good follow-up the control was not
foolproof. It enabled the practice to pinpoint the problem and take steps to
correct it. (An audit of lithium level control has since been conducted in the
practice using a similar methodology.)

(Dr Celia Teare and partners, Church St, Wantage, UK)

EXAMPLE 5 INADEQUATE CERVICAL SMEARS

Problem

A large proportion of cervical smears were reported to the practice as
inadequate, showing no endocervical cells.

Example 6   Use of chaperon   163

Data collection

The practice nurse kept a record of the smear results. The inadequate smear rate for different doctors in the practice varied from 22 per cent to 50 per cent.

Changes introduced

1. Greater care to be taken to take the smear from the squamo-columnar junction.
2. Fixative to be changed more regularly.
3. Ayre's spatulas to be used routinely.

Repeat data collection after a year

No doctor in the practice had above 26 per cent inadequate smears.

Repeat 5 years later

Inadequate smear rate for the practice was 17 per cent.

Conclusion

Audit may be embarrassing, but that is better than ignorance or apathy. The doctor originally least adequate now has figures better than the practice average. The practice did not set a target level of performance. Information from the laboratory about inadequate cervical smear rates for all local practices would help the practice to set itself such a target.

(Dr Richard Baker and partners, Leckhampton, Glos, UK)

EXAMPLE 6   USE OF CHAPERON

Problem

Doctors in a practice of four male doctors and one female doctor had worried about using a chaperon during intimate female examinations. A local newspaper article, coinciding with the annual reports of the Defence Societies about a female patient's allegations against her male doctor, brought these concerns to a head.

Data collection

The practice decided to audit patients' attitudes. A survey had been published showing that 75 per cent of 200 female patients questioned would like to be offered a chaperon, but only 6 per cent would accept if the examination were performed by their own doctor (Jones 1983).

With the help of a medical student the practice repeated the survey and attained similar results: 61 per cent of women would like to be offered a chaperon; 10 per cent would accept if the examination were performed by their own doctor; 21 per cent would accept if the examination were performed by another doctor.

Change introduced

1. Doctors should usually offer a chaperon to female patients.
2. The nurses would make arrangements for doctors to take patients to the nurse's room for examination if appropriate.

Conclusion

The doctors have perhaps over-reacted to the apparently reassuring findings, and the chaperoned intimate examination has become commonplace in the practice. This exemplifies that data alone cannot determine practice policy, it must be evaluated in conjunction with other feelings and evidence. Should an allegation be made against a doctor, the fact that sufficient concern has been shown for the matter to be audited would, the partners feel, count in their favour in any hearing.

(Dr Tom O'Dowd and partners, Calverton, Nottinghamshire, UK)

COMMENT

All these audits were carried out in the face of concern about the quality of some aspect of a practice's patient care. All produced change, resulting in improved care for patients, and improved security and confidence for the practice. They were all short and simple, and so could be repeated easily to monitor improvement and maintenance of improvement. Such an approach turns areas of uncertainty into areas of assured quality.

REFERENCES

Baker, R. (1990). Problem solving with audit in general practice. *British Medical Journal*, **300**, 378–80.
Jones, R. (1983). The use of chaperons by general practitioners. *Journal of the Royal College of General Practitioners*, **33**, 25–7.
Smith, C. (1991). Perfectly simple audits. *British Journal of General Practice*, **41**, 218.

15 Access, availability, and continuity

George Freeman

INTRODUCTION

General practice should offer both accessibility and continuity. The patient should find it an easy matter to see the doctor or other primary care team member at a convenient time. Care should be as continuous as required, that is consistent and uninterrupted. Since so much of general practice is based on interpersonal relationships, continuity tends to mean seeing the same person—any alternative implies a very high degree of communication between members of the care team, including the keeping of excellent records.

In the archetypal single-handed practice the practitioner was *available* for long hours and access was by coming and queuing. The patients always saw the same person, so *continuity* was only limited by the doctor's memory. Nowadays doctors work in groups with paramedical colleagues. Availability is negotiated through receptionists who operate an appointments system for most contacts with health team members. Although this was originally an attempt to eliminate queuing, appointments systems are also used to even out demand over a number of consulting sessions. The effect may limit both availability and continuity.

Continuity in the sense of a patient seeing the same doctor at every consultation has been one of the key features of general practice. The terms 'my doctor' and often 'my own doctor' are common parlance. Nevertheless, the rise of group practice has led to a reduction in continuity which can fall to relatively low levels. This is most likely to happen when patients have a 'free choice' of doctor combined with limited availability—such as a substantial commitment to a branch surgery, to teaching, or to work outside the practice.

Group practices tend to use either of two organizational systems—personal lists where patients normally see the doctor with whom they are registered, or alternatively a combined list where any doctor can be requested. The personal list system is in effect a number of single-handed appointment systems under one roof with some flexibility for sharing out peaks of demand. With the combined list system it is easier for receptionists to guide patients to less busy doctors. Most of the following audit suggestions apply particularly to combined list groups which are more common nowadays.

Availability and continuity tend to conflict with each other, more so if a practice is subconsciously using the appointments system to limit overall demand. The shorter the interval between booking time and requested appointment the more likely it is that the only available appointments will be with the least requested doctor. This may be a new partner or a trainee, or it may be a doctor who is less popular for some reason. Many patients prefer not to book appointments more than a day in advance (depending on coping skills, social class, etc.), whereas many doctors consider that only a minority of the problems brought to them need so short a timescale. The result is that when patients request appointments they may find their preferred doctor fully booked and have to negotiate either a different doctor at the time they wanted or else a longer wait for their preferred doctor.

Thus, it is necessary to distinguish between availability of appointments with any doctor and availability with a named doctor, in order that continuity is not sacrificed in pursuit of anonymous availability.

Demand in a health service which is free at the point of use can seem potentially limitless. Any appointment system, however well planned, can sometimes (or even often) seem stressful to those working it. The team of doctors and receptionists can gain much by finding out how good their system really is and whether they can feel proud of its quality. The methods outlined in this chapter have been developed and used by the author with practices in the Southampton area. The experience and results have been published (Freeman 1989; Freeman and Richards 1990).

AVAILABILITY

Setting a team standard

One fundamental *indicator* of availability is the number of free appointments available at any specified time with individuals and with the group as a whole. This can be measured for set intervals in advance, for example same day, next day, 3 days, 7 days, etc. These numbers have to be related to the daily totals of patients actually seen, in order for the practice to agree an appropriate *criterion*. For example, if a doctor sees an average of 30 patients each working day, then criteria of good availability could be set at 15 free appointments at the start of the same day, 35 within two days, and 25 available on the same day next week.

An alternative indicator of availability is the length of the intervals before, say, the next, tenth and 50th free appointments. The team can then agree a criterion in working days or half days. For instance, 'there should be less than two days before the next free appointment with each doctor'.

Even the best appointment system is beaten from time to time—this will show up as 'extras', 'fit-ins', or some other expression denoting a patient seen without an appointment. A large number of extras will indicate excessive pressure on the system. So a further indicator could be the number of extras seen each day: a criterion might be that this should be less then 10 per cent of all appointments.

At the other end of the spectrum the number of appointments never filled indicates inappropriate provision of service.

The next step in the audit cycle is to agree a *level of performance* for each criterion, in order to set a *target standard*. In the example of the doctor seeing 30 patients per working day and a criterion of 15 free appointments within 24 hours, the team might set a target that this criterion should be reached on 90 per cent of days audited. It is important at this stage not to be unrealistic. Ideally, a group of patients might be involved together with the team in setting the target, but certainly receptionists should have a good feel for its feasibility. If the target is to be met it is also important to think of confounding events, such as regular time out of the practice for teaching or clinical appointments and (half) days off duty—or even for attending a medical audit group.

Sampling and data collection (described for the first indicator only)

In this case recording is a simple matter. All that is needed is a table for assessing doctors and other clinical team members (for example treatment room sister) according to a planned system of recording sessions. In order to avoid bias it is essential to include both popular and less demanding days and times. In practice precise times are too complex to audit, but a session half day is a practical unit. It may be possible to sample every session in the week repeatedly, but it is probably enough to record one or two different sessions over, for example, a 10 week period in order to capture some of the random fluctuation in demand that seems to occur in most practices. Certainly, it will be important to assess each session during the week once or twice in order to be able to say something useful about the *distribution* of availability as well as the average.

Form I is suggested to record these data (Fig. 15.1). Collection of the data can be done by any properly briefed person. They will need a schedule of sessions and instructions for standardization, for example always record at the beginning of a session or the end of the previous one (for example, 11 am Saturday may be less stressful than 8.30 am Monday).

Once the data are collected someone must be responsible for collating and tabulating them. Each cell in the table is checked to see if the criterion set has been achieved and is then appropriately marked; marked cells in each column are then counted, 18 or more out of 20 will meet the 90 per cent target standard. The totals can then be charted as the *achieved standards* for individual doctors, all doctors, and treatment room sister.

Evaluation

All participants can now meet to *evaluate* the result. Congratulations are in order—to those collecting the data and to all those involved in planning and collations. The first audit cycle is nearly complete.

Date	Session	Dr A		Dr B		Dr C		Dr D		All doctors		Sister	
	*Next	2	4	2	4	2	4	2	4	2	4	2	4
Mon	am (week 1)												
	pm												
Tues	am												
	pm												
Wed	am												
	pm												
Thur	am												
	pm												
Fri	am												
	pm												
Mon	am (week 2)												
	pm												
Tues	am												
	pm												
Wed	am												
	pm												
Thur	am												
	pm												
Fri	am												
	pm												

* i.e. number of appointments free in the next 24 hours (2 sessions) and next 48 hours (4 sessions) recorded at the start of each session.

Fig. 15.1   Form I. Audit of availability of appointments with four doctors and one sister over 20 half-day sessions.

Agenda at team evaluation meeting

1. Presentation of achieved standard and comparison with the target.
2. Special and unforeseen factors — What went well and what not so well?
3. What does the achieved standard mean — Was the target appropriate? (too strict? too lax?) What other implications are there? In particular: Are enough appointments being offered in total? How many patients did not arrive? How many extras and unfilled appointments were there? What about telephone access to the doctors? A large team may find it helpful to divide into smaller groups to discuss these points.
4. What are we doing well — that we want to keep? What changes should be made to the appointment system?
5. How to repeat the cycle and do it better next time? Interval: 3, 6, 12 months?

CONTINUITY

While an audit of *availability* as already outlined may produce very useful pointers to improvement, it is probable that the receptionists (if not the doctors) will already have been aware of the extent of any problem in their everyday work. In the case of *continuity* an audit may be genuinely surprising to the team because the better established doctors will tend to think first of their continuity with regular, often older, patients while overlooking the extent to which younger patients, and children in particular, encounter a number of different team members.

Any practice with a computer system which records the provider of every consultation will be able to audit continuity from the date the system was fully installed and running smoothly. For most practices an initial approach can be a retrospective audit of patients' records, identifying the different doctors consulted by their handwriting. It is a great advantage if the continuation cards have been in date order for some years past, otherwise finding consecutive consultations on different cards may play havoc with the results.

Setting a team standard

A simple *indicator* is the percentage of each patient's contacts which are with the same doctor. This is the continuity index (Breslau and Reeb 1975) (originally defined in the USA as the usual provider continuity index, or UPCI), and it can be measured over a given period of time, or a given number of consultations, or a combination of the two. It is best to have a maximum time period—both to limit the work involved and to confine the audit to a time when all or most present team members have been in post. If the time period is too short, then too few consultations will be included to give a consistent picture. A reasonable compromise is two years, with a minimum of four consultations and a maximum of 12. This will exclude patients who consult infrequently and limit the work on high consulters to an acceptable level.

The *criterion* will be a chosen level of continuity index. Full 100 per cent personal continuity is impossible in the real world, and the highest published levels in a strict personal list practice—allowing for holidays and other absences—have approached 90 per cent (Marsh and Kaim-Caudle 1976). The theoretical minimum will be 33 per cent in a three partner practice which never employs any other doctor, 25 per cent in a four partner practice, and so on. Group practices with shared lists may wish to consider levels between 50 and 75 per cent depending on their beliefs and priorities. The team can then decide the proportion of patients who should meet the chosen criterion and so produce the *target standard*. There is clearly a trade-off here, there is no widely accepted criterion for continuity and the team might choose to set a target of, for example, 100 per cent achievement of a 60 per cent continuity index (in general 100 per cent achievement is desirable as a target level of performance, then *any* exceptions have to be explained). But some teams may prefer to aim for better then a 60 per cent continuity and accept an initially lower level of performance, for example 90 per cent achievement of 75 per cent continuity.

Sampling and data collection

The audit has already been limited to patients with a minimum of four consultations in two years. It is best to select patients from attendance lists rather than from the registered list, as these patients are both more relevant to the audit and more likely to be eligible for inclusion. As usual, large numbers give more reliable results, but an acceptable minimum might be ten patients per full-time equivalent doctor. Again it is best to spread data collection over a period of time, for example, one month, and to include sessions from all times of the week. Within sessions it is important not to take only the first ten eligible patients because these may have booked first—those towards the end, particularly any extras must also be included. The best way of giving all patients an equal chance of inclusion is to number them and then use a table of random numbers (see p. 62).

Eligible patients' records are then examined by someone familiar with the handwriting of all of the team and recorded on a table, such as Form II (Fig 15.2).

The team needs to decide whether to include home visits and out of hours calls, including the deputizing service where appropriate. Within the surgery, decisions need to be made about extra (i.e. unbooked) patients and also any clinics. It is helpful to go back to the original question—if the audit is about access to the same doctor at patient initiated consultations then these are the ones to be identified for data collection, so extras but not clinic patients must be included.

Evaluation

Again someone must be responsible for collecting and preparing the results for presentation to the team. It is well worth sorting the patients into age groups before adding up the figures. In this way it will be an easy matter to present the results for each age group separately—considerable differences in continuity index may be found. The index is calculated for each patient and then the proportion meeting the criterion worked out. It is also possible to calculate the mean (average) for each group and for the total. (Strictly speaking the indices of patients with widely differing consultation rates are not exactly comparable, but this can safely be ignored in practice. Truly exceptional patients—for example those seen every day for a month—can be excluded as long as they are not also forgotten.)

Date ....

Recorder ....

Patient: age or date of birth ...., sex M/F, registered doctor..................,

major problem(s) ....

| Consultations | | | Doctor | | | | | | (Problem) |
no	date	S/V/other	A	B	C	D	Tr	Loc	Remarks
Totals									

Total consultations x

Most with one doctor y with Dr B

Continuity index= y/x with Dr B

Patient's age-group (years) 0–14
                             15–44
                             45–64
                             65+

Fig. 15.2 Form II. Audit of continuity index.

Agenda at team evaluation meeting

Again, start with thanks and congratulations to those doing the work.

1. Presentation of achieved standard and comparison with the target.
2. Comments on data collection if these will assist interpretation.
3. Meaning of the achieved standard:
    —was the target appropriate?
    —was the result satisfactory?

—are the results surprising and what do they say about the service that has been offered?

—team members' impressions of patient opinion (receptionists and nurses may have heard many relevant comments).

4. Should the practice policy be changed at all either in its aim or in its implementation through the appointment system?

5. Plan to reassess if any changes are made.

(It is probably not sensible to repeat this exercise sooner than one year ahead.)

THE INTERACTION OF AVAILABILITY AND CONTINUITY

Availability and continuity are intimately linked. The first two audits will have produced some useful information about the level of availability, both for the group and for individuals, and about the resulting continuity of doctor that patients have received. This may well give sufficient information for the team to plan and implement change in the appointments system which can be audited in future cycles. Sometimes, however, such audits raise many more questions which need to be answered before effective change can be agreed upon. In this case it may be helpful to audit the 'sharp end' of the appointment system by monitoring the actual negotiation between patient and receptionist.

This audit needs an observer to record the patient/receptionist interaction while appointments are being made. It is therefore more difficult in requiring staff time (FHSAs may allocate resources to help practices do this sort of audit, either directly or through the MAAGs). Information from such observation may help team members to understand what is occurring, and point the way to workable solutions. For instance, the receptionists may be unwittingly encouraging more or less personal continuity, or apparent popularity of some partners may be real or may be due to high re-booking rates or to the lower availability of a part-time partner.

Setting team standards

It is always easier to satisfy a simple request. Thus, a patient requesting an appointment time or a particular doctor can better be accommodated than one requesting both.

In this audit there are several possible *indicators* which can be examined in one exercise. Nationally, there is little evidence on which to base criteria or agreed levels of performance. By collecting its own data within the practice the team may develop its own targets. The indicators and target standards listed here are just suggestions as starting points for discussion.

1. Indicator: the proportion of requests specifying: session only, doctor only, or doctor *and* session.

   Criterion: that patients should request a specific usual doctor.

Target level of performance: the team may decide that a high proportion (>80 per cent?) of requests should specify a doctor.

2. Criterion: that a request for a specific type of appointment should be successful (i.e. appointment made agrees with request).
   Target level of performance: >95 per cent? for session or doctor only
   >75 per cent? for session *and* doctor.

3. Indicator: the mean delay between request and agreed session. This indicator is perhaps the benchmark of the successful appointments system. Delays will probably vary between doctors if indicator 4 shows marked imbalance of requests.
   Criteria: Requests stipulating only the session should be satisfied within 24 hours (two sessions). Requests stipulating only the doctor should be satisfied within 48 hours (four sessions). Requests stipulating both session and doctor should be satisfied within 72 hours (six sessions).
   Target levels of performance: to be determined by the team, >80 per cent for each criterion?

4. Indicator: the doctor requested (if any). This indicator will give sensitive information about which doctors are most requested.
   Criterion: the maximum ratio of requests between different doctors (with equivalent shares) should not exceed, for example, 2:1 for the audit period without agreed special factors—such as a new partner starting up.
   Target level of performance: 100 per cent.

5. Indicator: the proportion of requests which are rebookings (made as the patient leaves the previous consultation) and with which doctors. This indicator combines patient factors, such as chronic illness and need for repeated follow-up, with doctor behaviour, since some doctors may suggest specific follow-up appointments much more often than their colleagues.
   Criterion: rebooked appointments during the audit period for any doctor should not exceed 50 per cent.
   Level of performance: 100 per cent. This target standard will involve repeated and constructive discussion between doctors and receptionists.

6. Indicator: the proportion of negotiations which end inconclusively. The proportion may represent a frustration index for the appointment system.
   Criterion: no negotiation for an appointment should end inconclusively.
   Target level of performance: <5 per cent?

7. Indicator: how many sessions ahead the patients are booking.
   Target standard: this is difficult. A criterion is difficult to define. For instance, some patients may be booking ahead if they know appointments are hard to get, others because they are on chronic disease monitoring and so legitimately need forward appointments. Data may well be necessary to increase understanding about the way patients have learned to use the appointments system. Even if no target is set at first, presentation of results may well lead to constructive discussion resulting in planning and target standard setting in the future.

Sampling and data collection

The receptionists need to feel comfortable with the observer (perhaps one of themselves) who will sit near the appointment desk and record the process of negotiation. More than 90 per cent of new appointments are made on the telephone in many practices, but the author's experience is that excellent data can be obtained by monitoring just the receptionists' share of the telephone negotiations. Occasionally clarification is necessary. Almost all appointments can be included, except at the busiest times on, for example, Monday morning. Again the appointment *session* is a practical unit which can be recorded just as either *am* or *pm* (including early evening).

Data are collected on Form III (Fig 15.3) and, as usual, it is necessary to record representative samples across the working week. Recording at quiet times may be clearly uneconomical for a separate observer, but the receptionists may be able to fill in the forms themselves at these times. In four Southampton group practices with list sizes exceeding 13 000 it was possible to record well over 500 appointment negotiations during 16 observation sessions none of which lasted more than two hours (Freeman 1989).

Evaluation

The result of this audit should 'explain' a number of the questions raised by the previous pair and need to be considered together with these.

Whether the target standards have been achieved will depend more than ever on how optimistic or realistic those were — since they were essentially arbitrary. More than one meeting may be needed. Within the meeting agenda the discussion will inevitably involve: what the team is really wanting to achieve; what it thinks is possible and appropriate; to what extent variation between doctors (demand for and behaviour of) is important to the whole picture and to the validity of underlying beliefs, such as 'there is no point in really offering enough appointments because this will only create more demand'.

Agenda of team evaluation meeting

1. Congratulations on achievement of a demanding audit.
2. Brief reminder of target standards and how these were chosen.
3. Presentation of standards achieved and comparison with targets.
4. Brief comment on data collection methods. Anecdotes may be plentiful, most of these are probably best postponed until the main issues have been agreed (see 6).
5. Meaning of the achieved standards under the following headings: Do patients' wishes appear to be reasonable — are they as expected? Is the team providing the overall service level it wishes? Are there enough appointments

Date..............................

Recorder.......................

Recep tionist	Request			Offer		Outcome	Comment
	time	(1) Doctor (2)*	Day/ session	Doctor/time (1)	Doctor/time (2)	Agreed appointment	

Note special features of session: (doctors absent, influenza epidemic, etc.)

* i.e. first requested doctor and second choice (if any).

Fig. 15.3 Form III. Audit of appointment requests and outcomes.

overall? Are there particular problems: for example, difficult times in the week, demand for particular doctors or for 'lady doctors', is any imbalance in demand for individual partners explained by different rebooking rates?
6. If the answer to any of these is yes then change must be sought, either in what service is provided, or in how patients are encouraged to use it, or both.
7. Agree a preliminary agenda for changes and realistic targets for future performance.
8. Appoint one or more working groups to plan specific changes.
9. Timetable for working groups to report back to a future meeting to agree: implementation of changes, target standards and timing for the next audit.

CONCLUSION

These audits should give the team much better insight into their performance in a crucial area of practice. If enough teams can get a good feel for how their appointment systems really work then general practice will be in a much better position to say to the public and to the government what medical service can realistically be offered. Appointment systems are essential to allow primary care teams to plan their service properly, but they effectively conceal the kind of rationing that has to be applied to a system which is free at the time of use. Practices depend on patients not making unreasonable demands, while half fearing that they will, but these demands may often be fashioned by previous experience. Audit enables the team to understand what experience the patients are getting and so make change more relevant and effective.

FURTHER AUDITS

There are clearly other ways of auditing this area, in particular surveying patients' opinions directly or investigating how much a patient's perceived urgency is related to the content of the subsequent consultation as judged by the doctor or other team member.

Auditing patients' opinions by interviewing them in the waiting room or by distributing questionnaires may give reliable information. This type of audit is discussed fully in Chapter 16. It is especially valuable to see whether the practice's perception of good availability and continuity is reflected by patients' views and satisfaction. It can also be very useful if a major change is envisaged outside the practice's and the patients' current experience.

Examining critical events can also illuminate the workings of the appointment system. Either patients can be asked to relate particular experiences on visiting the surgery (p. 183); or the practice team can meet to examine particular days when the system seemed to break down, or particular episodes when one patient may have had especial problems. This approach is discussed in Chaper 13.

Studying the outcome of appointment requests may be a very useful further exercise to supplement the three audits outlined in this chapter. This could be developed to help receptionists learn what really happens in consultations and relate this to their own work experience. Provided such learning is used to improve receptionists' ability to teach patients to use their system well this may bring important benefits — because real progress is only made when receptionists can do more than just offer an undifferentiated appointment with a doctor. A well-informed receptionist should not be a barrier, but a facilitator in improved primary medical care.

REFERENCES

Breslau, N. and Reeb, K. G. (1975). Continuity of care in a university-based practice. *Journal of Medical Education*, **50**, 965–9.

Freeman, G. K. (1989). Receptionists, appointment systems and continuity of care. *Journal of the Royal College of General Practitioners*, **39**, 145–7.

Freeman, G. K. and Richards, S. C. (1990). How much personal care in four group practices? *British Medical Journal*, **301**, 1028–30.

Marsh, G. and Kaim-Caudle, P. (1976). Team care in general practice. Croom Helm, London.

16 Assessment of patients' views in primary care

Ray Fitzpatrick

The new contract requires family practitioner committees to carry out surveys to assess patients' views of their general practice services. At the same time it is now expected that patients' views should be included in medical audit in primary care. This chapter considers some of the methods involved. Whilst indicating the potential value and scope of consumer surveys, the chapter also discusses the potential pitfalls and problems that are frequently encountered.

REASONS FOR ASSESSING PATIENTS' VIEWS

First, it is important briefly to clarify the different reasons why the importance of patients' views has been so much emphasized in recent policy documents about the health service. One factor is the growing acceptance that the patient provides an important indicator of the quality of care. Indeed, in many aspects of primary care, such as the accessibility of the practice, the receptionist's manner, or the availability of out of hours care, the patient's views may be one of the main indicators of quality.

A second factor is the widespread view that patients as citizens are entitled to express their views about services that are publicly funded. It will also allow patients to participate in the shape and direction of health services that they receive.

A third view is that patient satisfaction is actually an objective of health care, and may therefore be used as an outcome measure alongside morbidity and survival. Not everyone finds this view acceptable. Some argue that consumers may give us important feedback about the *processes* of care, how well services are provided, but not of *outcomes* in terms of benefits to health. They would cite the problem of the patient who is satisfied with care that in medical terms may be unhelpful or indeed harmful. However, whether or not patient satisfaction is an outcome measure, there is clear evidence that satisfaction has important effects on outcomes. Satisfied patients are more likely to follow their recommended treatments, re-attend for further treatment, and stay with their current general practitioner. Moreover, there is growing evidence that satisfaction is positively related to improvements in health status (Fitzpatrick 1991).

POTENTIAL PROBLEMS

Are patients' views threatening?

There are a number of concerns often expressed about the idea of carrying out a survey of patients' views. One common misapprehension is that the survey will uncover demoralizing levels of dissatisfaction. However, in most surveys of primary care, the majority of patients—typically 80–85 per cent—express positive satisfaction with primary care. In one study (Rashid *et al.* 1989), 50 patients from each of five general practitioners were asked to state their views about their consultations. The doctors were asked to assess the same consultations with parallel questionnaires. It emerged that the doctors were more critical than the patients with regard to various aspects of the consultations. Health professionals may overestimate the extent of problems perceived by patients.

Are patients' views reliable?

A very different suspicion is that patients' views will be ill-considered and superficial. Undoubtedly there is evidence that patients' judgements about the professional competence or value of medical treatment from a general practitioner can be influenced by other criteria, such as perceptions of his or her interpersonal manner. The problem may arise from questionnaires that are poorly designed containing questions that are too vague to allow patients to distinguish their views on different aspects of family practice services. Doubts about the consistency and stability of patients' views are, unfortunately, rarely addressed in surveys. What in technical terms is referred to as the reliability of an instrument can be examined in two ways. First, the extent of agreement obtained between two different administrations of a questionnaire can be measured. The small number of, mainly American, studies that have examined consistency over time have been encouraging. However, one of the few British general practice-based studies found a significant decline in patient satisfaction on a number of different aspects of a consultation one week later, compared with views expressed immediately after the consultation (Savage and Armstrong 1990).

An alternative approach is to establish that a questionnaire has internal reliability—i.e. that questionnaire items about similar issues produce consistent answers. The principle of internal reliability can be illustrated by a patient satisfaction questionnaire recently developed for use in general practice (Baker 1990). A questionnaire was developed by a number of different methods which resulted in a number of items that had been shown to be unambiguous and produce a range of responses. At this point, and in further cycles to improve the questionnaire, the items were analysed statistically to identify and eliminate items that did not produce answers consistent with any others. By this approach, four separate scales or groups of questions were produced assessing views in relation to the following areas: general satisfaction, professional care, depth of relationship, and perceived time. The four scales were internally reliable, in the sense that individual questionnaire items correlated or agreed with other items in the same scale covering the same issue. Thus, for example, respondents were asked to say to what extent they agreed with the following two items:

1. This doctor was very careful to check everything when examining me.
2. This doctor examined me very thoroughly.

The main reason for this overlap between items is that it is considered that any question has a certain amount of measurement error in terms of whether it accurately assesses the underlying attitude or view. A number of related items, if they are shown to correlate with each other, increase the accuracy with which the view is measured. In this case, the two items just quoted were found to correlate with each other and to contribute to a scale of seven items in all that measured the extent of satisfaction with the doctor's professional care. These items are then treated as a single scale and scored as such.

Are questionnaires valid?

The more challenging problem that needs to be addressed is whether questionnaires actually measure the views that they are intended to measure — in technical terms the problem of *validity*. In practical terms it is quite difficult ever to give a definite answer to this question. However, it is worth drawing the reader's attention to research studies (of a kind probably beyond the scope of routine audit) which have elegantly shown that patients' views as expressed in questionnaires do relate to particular aspects of their health care experiences. So, for example, Stiles *et al.* (1979) tape-recorded the consultations of 19 doctors and quantified various aspects of their approaches to taking the patient's history and style of communication. Patients completed a satisfaction questionnaire after leaving the consultation. When the two sources of data were analysed together, patient satisfaction was found to be positively associated with a particular measure from the tapes that assessed whether the doctor encouraged patients to describe their problem in their own terms. The authors concluded that patients who had been given an ample opportunity to give their own view of their problem were more likely to feel the doctor had listened and understood their problem. For us, however, the important point was a methodological one — that it was possible to show systematic relations between views expressed in a questionnaire and aspects of care independently assessed. Such studies are one method of *validating* a questionnaire.

It is unlikely that such detailed investigations would be feasible for most people considering measuring patient satisfaction in the context of medical audit. Nevertheless, it is still possible to examine some aspects of the validity of questionnaires or interviews. One method is to examine *content validity*. Do the items in the questionnaire appear adequately to assess the issues for which they are intended? This can best be done by obtaining the widest possible range of views about the content of the questionnaire. Thus patients, receptionists, health visitors, and individuals with as diverse a range of experiences of health care as possible may be invited to comment on the content and coverage of proposed instruments.

Is satisfaction a single entity?

Reference has been made to the concept of patient satisfaction. All too frequently, surveys in general practice are conducted with a view that this is a unitary phenomenon. The problem with this approach is that patients hold distinct views with regard to different aspects of their health care. Thus, patients may have views with regard to the friendliness and courtesy of surgery staff; the ease of access to appointments; the quality of medical care; the availability of after hours care, etc. In this sense, patients' views are multi-dimensional and cannot sensibly be reduced to an overall global score for satisfaction. Statistical analysis will generally show the results of a questionnaire of patients' views to comprise different distinct dimensions. Thus, when Baker carried out a survey using the patient satisfaction questionnaire that he had developed, four different factors emerged, as described above. The problem with using a single global measure of satisfaction is that it is very likely to mask differences of views with regard to different aspects of care.

METHODS OF OBTAINING PATIENTS' VIEWS

Questionnaires

There are a range of alternative methods of gathering patients' views. At one extreme is the method that most readily comes to mind — the *fixed format, self-completed questionnaire*. The simplest form of this type of questionnaire involves a series of questions of the form:

Are you satisfied with the following aspects of this practice?
1. *Making an appointment to see the doctor: Yes, No, Don't know.*
2. *Waiting room facilities: Yes, No, Don't know.*

(Adapted from Steven and Douglas 1986)

The main advantages of this method compared with an interview are that it is relatively inexpensive and straightforward to gather and process the information. Also, the information is gathered in a standardized fashion that appears to avoid any possible interviewer effects that might bias results. However, there are important limitations. It is difficult within the format of a questionnaire to explore more complex views or to establish the grounds or reasoning behind patients' statements. Similarly, an interviewer is better placed to clarify any misunderstanding the respondent may have about a question. However, careful attention to questionnaire development can overcome some of the claimed limitations of fixed choice questions. A more serious limitation of the questionnaire is that the content and focus is more firmly determined by the investigator; a fixed format questionnaire leaves very little scope for the repondent to raise issues important to him or her but not covered by the questionnaire. Again, it is possible to exaggerate the disadvantages of the questionnaire in this respect. If a questionnaire has been carefully piloted, it should cover most aspects of a topic that concerns patients. A related difficulty with a questionnaire is that it treats all aspects or topics as of equal importance, whereas for the patient, some particular experience or problem may be of paramount importance.

One possible compromise is to include in a fixed format questionnaire some *open-ended questions*. Respondents may, for example, be asked to say which aspects of a general practice they found most annoying, without being given a range of response categories. It allows the respondent some scope for conveying views not covered by the questionnaire. However, it has to be kept in mind that the information gathered in this way will eventually have to be coded and that coding free-format answers is particularly time-consuming. With a mailed questionnaire, the respondent has no opportunity to infer the kinds of answers required from an open-ended question, and this may make the task of completing such questions more difficult and indeed frustrating. For reasons of acceptability and economy in processing results, such open-ended questions in a self-completed questionnaire tend to be kept to a minimum.

Interviews

Interviews are considered to have a number of advantages over, for example, postal questionnaires. The interviewer may establish rapport, and thus make it more likely that the respondent completes the task. As already indicated, an interview allows for clarification of ambiguities in questions and sensitivity to the differential importance or salience of issues. It is also possible to cover more topics in the course of an interview than with a postal questionnaire. The disadvantages of an interview are that it is more costly and time consuming to gather the information. Interviews are unlikely to succeed without basic training of staff in both interviewing skills and the specific objectives of the current study. Interviews have a number of different formats. Most frequently they involve the same basic *fixed format* as a self-completed questionnaire and only differ in being personally administered.

Interviews may also be of an *unstructured format*, in which respondents have the maximum opportunity to assert and discuss views in their own terms. This approach is considered more likely to be sensitive to patients' own agenda (Fitzpatrick and Hopkins 1983). However, the effort involved in the content analysis of such interviews is very considerable. A particularly detailed study was carried out of patients' views of out of hours care, in which patients were interviewed and the interviews tape recorded (Bollam *et al.* 1988). Ratings were subsequently made of patients' views from the tape-recordings. However, the study produced no more variation of views than might be expected from more conventional and less costly methods. Careful thought is needed about the additional data expected to be gained from more in-depth but more costly means of gathering and assessing patients' views.

A compromise format is the *structured interview* interspersed with items on key issues in which respondents are asked *open-ended questions*. Thus, for example, in an otherwise structured interview to obtain views of general practice in inner London (Curtis 1987), respondents were asked without prompts to say what types of improvements to surgery premises and facilities they would like to see; the qualities in their general practice they most appreciated; and again the qualities they felt a general practice ought to have but which were lacking in their own. The investigators regarded the results of these spontaneous items as particularly revealing of more salient issues to respondents.

A particular variant of semi-structured interview relying on *critical incident technique* (CIT) has recently been developed for use in assessing patients' views. The method essentially requires a trained interviewer to facilitate the respondent in giving a free-form narrative of a particular episode or incident, for example a particular visit to the surgery. Content analysis is used to delineate the different key steps or stages in the narratives of a sample, for example, arranging the appointment, getting to the surgery, the period of waiting in the surgery, etc. The primary objective is to record salient positive and negative comments in relation to each step or stage. Advocates of the approach say that whilst the method permits a calculation of the ratio of positive to negative comments for different experiences or aspects of a consultation, this calculation is secondary to the actual content of comments (Gau *et al.* 1989). The narrative form of interview encourages people to recall experiences in quite graphic form and the results may have a more vivid impact on audit than the reporting of percentages dissatisfied with this or that aspect of general practice. Thus, CIT methodology in one study (Gau *et al.* 1989) produced considerable variation in views about out of hours care. The following quotation from one respondent interviewed gives some indication of the vividness and value of this approach for audit purposes:

My daughter was ill one time and I rang up the duty doctor for some advice. He was very unhelpful—I thought he was irritable, condescending and very patronising—that isn't helpful at the best of times, but when you are worried it is very bad.

Good qualitative material may provide just as useful feedback for the purposes of provoking critical appraisal of practice.

CONDUCTING A SURVEY

Before any formal survey of patients' views is carried out, certain steps need to be taken. If resources are available a *pre-pilot* study is invaluable. This would normally involve exploratory unstructured interviews with some patients in which every opportunity is given to respondents to raise issues that might otherwise be neglected in the main survey. Remember that one of the main limitations of a structured interview or questionnaire that is likely to be the method of choice in the main survey is that respondents have little or no chance to express views outside the range determined by those who design the survey. The pre-pilot is an important opportunity to overcome this constraint.

Having decided on the topics to be covered and devised in a questionnaire, the instrument must be subjected to a *pilot survey*. This is the opportunity to establish whether the questionnaire as a whole is acceptable; whether individual questionnaire items are acceptable and easily understood, and whether the distribution of answers is informative. It is also possible to test alternative versions of a question or set of questions, or alternative forms of presentation.

SAMPLING

The overall objective in drawing a sample is to obtain the views of a group of respondents who are as likely as possible to be representative of the population whose views are wanted. The majority of general practice studies are based on patients actually attending surgery who are asked to complete the questionnaire immediately before or after their consultation. This may make sense when the focus of the questionnaire is the consultation episode. It would not be a satisfactory method if views of all of the patients in the practice were required, since recent attenders would be over-represented. More specific sources may be considered depending on the subject. Thus, in order to study patients' views of out of hours care, Bollam *et al.* (1988) required a number of general practices and the local deputizing agencies to record details of all out of hours calls over a specified period. Their sample was obtained from this sub-group of patients. Having identified the target population which will constitute the *sampling frame*, it is absolutely essential to obtain the highest possible response rate, since there is always the suspicion that non-respondents are more likely to be dissatisfied. The approach of sampling from attenders has the advantage that response rates are very high, typically in the range 90—95 per cent. This compares with mailed surveys which often fall below 50 per cent. Follow-up questionnaires to non-respondents will raise the response rate but, of course, the ability to do this depends on knowing the identities of respondents and non-respondents.

The method of deriving a sample also needs to be decided. The most common method in studies of general practice attenders is to take consecutive attenders in a given time period. This may be a problem if too short a time period is used, so that certain types of attenders are under-represented. An alternative is the quota sample, in which the investigator sets predetermined targets of numbers of patients in terms of age, sex, or other characteristics. A more elaborate method is to use *random sampling*. Thus, Savage and Armstrong (1990) used a random number generator to select patients in advance from patients attending the surgery.

Questionnaires need clearly to guarantee the confidentiality of respondents' answers. This is most easily done if no means of identifying individuals is used. Whilst appropriate to many purposes, anonymity cannot be employed if it is intended to follow-up non-respondents. Some surveys use hidden markers on the questionnaire which, whilst reassuring respondents of the anonymity of answers, actually enable non-respondents to be identified. Such deceptions clearly raise ethical issues that may make the practice unacceptable. If resources permit, it is advisable to have an independent organization carry out the survey. In this way, respondents may be encouraged to be more candid in expressing their views. Thus, general practice surveys may be conducted by the local Community Health Council (Williamson 1989) or by a university department (Baker 1990).

USES OF PATIENT SURVEYS

A single survey

Patients' views are most commonly obtained in simple 'one-off' surveys. The intention is to obtain descriptive evidence of those aspects of a general practice which give rise to satisfaction or dissatisfaction. The survey is thus used to provide feedback to a practice and is potentially a means of identifying problems in the provision of care.

Analytical uses

Occasionally the patient satisfaction survey has been used more ambitiously in a general practice context. Thus, patient satisfaction scores may be used as an outcome measure in a study design in which patients are randomly allocated to two different styles of communication (for example, 'doctor-centred' versus 'patient centred') (Savage and Armstrong 1990) or different lengths of consultation time (Ridsdale *et al.* 1989). Alternatively, instead of imposing variation in the form of a randomized trial, sometimes it is possible to examine the effects on patient satisfaction of varying forms of general practice that occur naturally. Thus, consultations will tend to vary in the degree to which they are patient-centred. Henbest and Stewart (1990) recorded and rated a range of consultations in this respect and related this information to patient satisfaction.

Howie *et al.* examined effects upon patient satisfaction of naturally occurring lengths of consultations measured across a number of general practitioners (Howie *et al.* 1991).

Monitoring change over time

To date it is unusual to see views assessed repeatedly, to assess changes over time. An exception is the work of Steven and Douglas (1986), who were concerned with the value of feeding back patients' views to their doctors. They used a simple 21 item satisfaction questionnaire (items illustrated above) to obtain patients' views about a number of different practices. Then the general practitioners were randomly assigned either to receive or not to receive feedback in terms of results from their patients' questionnaires. Six months later another sample of patients from both groups of doctors were asked to complete identical questionnaires, in order to assess whether feedback to one group of general practitioners resulted in any changes to the practice that would influence patient satisfaction. Individual doctors in the feedback group made changes in areas such as access by telephone and lengths of appointment, and patient dissatisfaction was markedly reduced at the re-test in these areas. The results were not significant. However, the majority of general practitioners felt the procedure had been valuable as an exercise in audit.

PROBLEMS IN INTERPRETATION

One important reason why this study did not reach significance in detecting effects of feedback upon patient satisfaction is that for most questionnaire items, less than 10 per cent of patients expressed dissatisfaction. Indeed, as already pointed out, 85 per cent of patients express positive satisfaction in questionnaires. One of the reasons for this pattern is that patients are reluctant to express negative views. Undoubtedly, lack of variability in views does make this method difficult to use in the cycle of audit. It also means that quite large numbers of patients need to be recruited to identify the effects upon patient satisfaction of specific processes of care. This emphasizes the role of qualitative approaches, such as critical incident technique, in providing material for critical appraisal of practice.

An additional consideration when attempting to obtain patients' views for purposes of audit is that patients' background characteristics may have an important influence upon answers. In particular, older patients tend to express more positive satisfaction. Other variables that may also have an effect are social class, education, gender, psychological well-being, and health status. The possible confounding effects of such variables need always to be examined before drawing inferences from any survey not conducted with randomization.

Medical audit has tended to focus upon such data as treatments, investigations, organizational arrangements, and referral rates. There has been a long tradition in general practice of assessing patients' views, but it has been viewed as a distinct and separate exercise from mainstream audit. General practice is now more explicitly required to take account of the patient's perspective. The main message of this chapter is that the same care and attention to method and interpretation is required in this field as in other areas of audit covered by this volume.

REFERENCES

Baker, R. (1990). Development of a questionnaire to assess patients' satisfaction with consultations in general practice. *British Journal of General Practice*, **40**, 487–90.
Bollam, M., McCarthy, M., and Modell, M. (1988) Patients' assessments of out of hours care in general practice. *British Medical Journal*, **296**, 829–32.
Curtis, S. (1987) The patient's view of general practice in an urban area. *Family Practice*, **4**, 200–206.
Fitzpatrick, R. (1991). Patient satisfaction surveys — important general considerations. *British Medical Journal*, **302**, 887–9.
Fitzpatrick, R. and Hopkins, A. (1983). Problems in the conceptual framework of patient satisfaction research. *Sociology of Health and Illness*, **5**, 297–311.
Gau, D., Pryce Jones, M., and Tipins, D. (1989). Satisfactory progress. *Health Service Journal*, **30 Nov.**, 1464–5.
Henbest, R. and Stewart, M. (1990). Patient-centredness in the consultation. 2: does it really make a difference? *Family Practice*, **7**, 28–33.
Howie, K., Porter, A., Heney, D., and Hopton, J. (1991). Long to short consultation ratio: a proxy measure of quality of care for general practice. *British Journal of General Practice*, **41**, 48–54.
Rashid, A., Forman, W., Jagger, C., and Mann, R. (1989). Consultations in general practice: a comparison of patients' and doctors' satisfaction. *British Medical Journal*, **299**, 1015–16.
Ridsdale, L., Carruthers, M., Morris, R., and Ridsdale, J. (1989). Study of the effect of time availability on the consultation. *Journal of the Royal College of General Practitioners*, **39**, 488–91.
Steven, I. and Douglas, R. (1986). A self contained method of evaluating patient dissatisfaction in general practice. *Family Practice*, **3**, 14–19.
Stiles, W., Putnam, S., Wolf, M., and James, S. (1979). Interaction exchange structure and patient satisfaction with medical interviews. *Medical Care*, **17**, 667–81.
Savage, R. and Armstrong, D. (1990). Effect of a general practitioner's consulting style on patients' satisfaction: a controlled study. *British Medical Journal*, **301**, 968–70.
Williamson, V. (1989). Patients' satisfaction with general practitioner services: a survey by a community health council. *Journal of the Royal College of General Practitioners*, **39**, 452–5.

17 Auditing teamwork

Karen Munro

One of the major themes of this book is that the delivery of most of the services in general practice depends on the contribution of members of different disciplines in the primary health care team, and that those involved in delivering the service should also be involved in auditing its quality. If this reveals areas in which the service could be improved, this may be related to the quality and effectiveness of the process of teamwork. This chapter will explore the audit of teamwork itself.

CHOOSING THE TOPIC

The link between the quality of teamwork and the quality of the service provided has been documented more fully in industrial settings than in primary health care (Adair 1986).

Teamwork acts by:

1. Ensuring that staff skills are used in the most appropriate combinations to deliver quality services in the most cost-effective manner, thus improving resource management.
2. Improving staff morale due to a sense of achievement and the positive feelings generated about working in a cohesive team environment. Improvements in morale tend to generate increased levels of confidence and a greater willingness among team members to undertake new challenges and to innovate.
3. Producing improved working relationships and a greater amount of understanding about roles and responsibilities amongst team members, thus helping to reduce professional rivalries and territorial disputes common between health care professionals.
4. Increasing patient choice by extending the range of health professionals available for consultation.

A further reason for considering an audit of teamwork is that many of the processes involved, clarifying values, defining roles, examining the contribution of different team members, and exploring the way that the team actually works, can all contribute to team building and improving the quality of the teamwork.

Before embarking on such an audit it is crucial to resolve some issues that strongly influence the whole approach of teams and teamwork in any practice. First, how does the practice define a team, and in what circumstances should a team approach be employed? There are many definitions of teamwork, and some practices believe that loose coalitions and general co-operation between members of the practice constitutes teamwork. Essentially, an effective team is a number of individuals who have need of each other's skills and who work closely together in order to accomplish a shared task which could not be undertaken by one person alone, or which could only be completed by using a team.

Many primary health care 'teams' are in fact a network of smaller groups, each of which may or may not work effectively as a team.

Some of these groups may be from a single discipline, for example, the partners, the community nurses, or the reception staff. Some practices have, however, developed multidisciplinary teams to develop and manage particular aspects of a practice's work. This has the advantage of creating groups which are of an effective size and do not involve all the members of the team in every meeting or activity.

The second question is whether groups already existing in the practice could work better together as a team, or does the practice need to create new teams to deal with certain tasks?

Finally, how much do practice leaders truly value teamwork as an integral part of the working in the practice? This is a vital issue as the actual degree of importance attributed to teamwork by influential members of the practice will determine whether teams are established and supported. Values and beliefs about ways in which teams ought to be structured and operate can also have a direct bearing on the potential success or failure of teamwork.

GETTING STARTED

There are a number of steps on the path between a practice recognizing that it wishes to develop its teamwork and the creation of effective teams. These are shown in the list below. If the team has agreed that it wishes to audit its teamwork performance separately from its performance in achieving tasks, then, it must decide whether it wishes to audit every aspect of the teamwork process or to address only those features which create obvious or suspected problems.

1. Identify practice priorities.
2. Specify areas of work requiring a team approach.
3. Create a team:
    (a) define team task
    (b) choose skill mix
    (c) establish membership
    (d) identify leader.
4. Clarify values.
5. Agree roles and responsibilities.

6. Establish framework for teamworking:
    (a) meetings and organization
    (b) communication
    (c) decision-making
    (d) criteria for audit.
7. Review
    (a) task achievement
    (b) process of teamwork

It is important to agree the amount of time the group of individuals is prepared to commit together to convert the group into a team. One indicator of the health of a team can be the amount of time that the team spends together and true teamwork depends on shared team time.

Much of the success of teamwork appears to depend on intangible forces, such as team spirit, morale, and enthusiasm, which are difficult to measure in an objective fashion. Much of the data relating to team effectiveness is therefore subjective, relying on the feelings or perceptions of team members about how well they think their team is performing. As a first stage the practice may wish to review the series of questions shown in the list below, which are related to the steps involved in team building. These may be considered during a review meeting, incorporated into a questionnaire to team members, or form part of the agenda of regular team meetings, particularly if specific problems have been identified.

1. Based on your assessment of progress with the team task, do you think you have the right mix of people and skills within your team?
2. Is team size hindering your progress? For example, is it too small and therefore of insufficient number to cover all the functions, or too large and therefore has difficulty reaching any decisions?
3. It the team leader leading? How comfortable are you with the leadership style in your team?
4. Are your team objectives clear and are they still relevant? Are you making any progress toward achieving them?
5. Do your team members have shared values about teamwork and team organization? Does there seem to be a lot of conflict between members about the right way to operate as a team?
6. Are you having any problems with the team organization and its working systems?
7. Are you happy with the way you take decisions as a team? Are many of your team decisions lost and not acted upon?
8. Does everybody in the team seem to care about each other's roles or is role overlap and confusion common?
9. Have you set up any systems to monitor your progress and performance in relation to team task? Are these systems working and if not why not?

The answers to these questions can then lead to more focused discussion identifying the reasons why team members feel there are problems in particular areas, what their criteria for effectiveness would be, what further information is required to clarify the problem, and what plans can be made to resolve it. In other words, these questions can be the starting point of operating the audit cycle in relation to a particular aspect of teamwork in the practice.

It is important, however, that irrespective of whether it is the teamwork or a team task that is the focus of this discussion all the team members should be involved in it. There is no doubt that those doing the work have the best understanding of the demands and constraints inherent in their work and the keenest insight into any associated problems and are thus most eligible to make recommendations for change to improve performance.

Following these discussions the team may then wish to audit particular aspects of the teamwork process and there are a number of approaches and tools which have been found to be helpful.

CLARIFYING VALUES

An exercise in clarifying values to discover real attitudes about teamwork is an essential precursor to improving teamwork itself. This may be particularly useful when teams are aware of poor teamwork but are unable to articulate any specific cause.

A questionnaire that could be used to stimulate discussion of values is shown in the appendix to this chapter. The discussions that this can provoke include:

Equality

1. Does 'equal treatment' mean equal status within the team or equality on the basis that all contributions to team purpose are valued equally and treated seriously?
2. Do those team members or leaders espousing equality 'live the value', i.e. do they practice what they preach?

Information and power

1. Is information sharing poor?
2. If so, is any deficiency due to poor communication, unwillingness to share or judgements by the information holders about what other team members need to know?

Team objectives

1. Does team objective setting need to be formalized?

Authority

1. Who has authority inside or outside the team?
2. Is respect automatic or must it be earned?

Winning/losing

1. Does competition exist between the members of your team?
2. How does it manifest itself?
3. How does competition exist between your team and others within the practice?
4. Would collaboration be more productive?

Trust

1. Building trust based on mutual respect takes time. How far has your team progressed towards achieving trust?

Risk taking

1. The degree of comfort with risk taking in any organization (not with patient care, but with innovative ideas for team organization, etc.) is related to the organization's attitude to failure or errors.
2. If the organization frowns upon errors or penalizes failure, its members will tend to avoid risks in the form of innovation or role extension. What is the attitude to mistakes in your team?

Professional standing

1. Do feelings of awe or lack of security in one's own value in the team diminish involvement of some team members?

Openness

1. Do some team members find it easier to be open and frank about opinions than others?
2. Is it linked to their perception of their status in the team?

Leadership

1. Good leaders make for effective teams.
2. The role of leader can be conferred, the recognition and acceptance of leader status needs to be earned.

Any of these issues may emerge naturally during discussions, but equally well may be deliberately avoided, particularly if they are problem areas.

TEAM ROLES

Members of a team occupy roles by virtue of their professional training and skills, and the extent to which they can use those skills may be influenced by the structure within which they have to operate. An essential ingredient of teamwork is that members of a team each know how they can contribute to the common task and the contribution that other team members do or could make.

A valuable exercise is to invite all the members of the team to write down their understanding of the skills, the functions, and the constraints of each of the other team members and to identify overlaps with other team roles. This may be considered in relation to each individual's total work, but the ensuing discussion may sometimes be more productive and fruitful if the questions are answered in relation to one particular task of the team. This exercise in role clarification is an essential step in planning practice activities, for example, health promotion, management of chronic conditions, or care of the elderly.

Another way to examine roles is to consider the contribution that each member of a team makes to the process of its work. Belbin (1981) studied the different roles that group members could perform and the effectiveness of groups which contained different mixes of individuals. These roles are shown in Table 17.1.

The essential conclusion from these studies was that teams which contained people who were performing each of these roles were much more effective than groups that either lacked particular roles or contained a large number of people trying to occupy the same role. Using a questionnaire it is possible for

Table 17.1 *Belbin's classification of team roles*

Role	Description
The plant	The member with a fluent mind and divergent thinking who creates new ideas.
The shaper	Looks for patterns in the team's discussions in an effort to unite ideas and push the team towards decisions and actions.
The monitor/evaluator	An analytical thinker. Able to assess accurately the feasibility of proposed solutions and actions.
The company worker	Has the capacity to convert decisions into practical lines of action.
The resource investigator	Has outside contacts and information, and the ability to stimulate the team and prevent stagnation.
The finisher	Galvanizes the team into action, and is concerned with overcoming things that may go/have gone wrong.
The team worker	Offers support and help to individual members and builds up the social character and effectiveness of the group.

individuals to identify their preferred roles and also the other roles that they are capable of occupying.

The importance of this approach to a team is in negotiating each member's contribution and sometimes in recruiting new members to perform roles which are missing. Some of the roles that Belbin describes, for example the plant or the shaper, have a higher profile than others and a further advantage to a team of undertaking this exercise is to acknowledge the essential contribution that all its members, including team workers and completer finishers, make to a team's effectiveness.

TEAM ORGANIZATION

Even if a team has clarified its values and the roles of its members, the way it actually works may still not be effective. Problems frequently lie in three areas: team meetings, systems of communication, and the process of decision making. The topics that could be discussed in each area are outlined below.

Team meetings

1. Establish purpose of meetings.
2. Agree frequency; duration; required attendance rate by members; venue; and preferred time of day to meet.
3. Details of agenda, i.e. format; circulation procedure; person responsible for constructing the agenda; and the contribution expected from other team members.
4. Details of minutes, i.e. how team decisions and team members responsible for actioning decisions will be recorded; circulation procedure; identifying person responsible for recording the minutes.

Communication systems

1. Decide which information will be transmitted verbally, and what needs to be in writing.
2. Allocate primary responsibility to individual team members to liaise with specific groups or individuals outside the team.

Decision-making systems

1. Type of system to be used to reach decisions in team meetings, for example majority vote, consensus, etc.
2. Establish circumstances under which team members (all or only those delegated to do so) would be authorized to 'speak' for the team, and to take decisions on their behalf.
3. Agree mechanism for monitoring the use of the agreed systems.

Criteria for auditing this aspect of teamwork will vary considerably depending upon the rigour and amount of detailed investigation of the type of audit to be undertaken, but the criteria should always be linked to the stated objectives about teamwork process.

Once criteria are agreed, information can be obtained either from subjective feedback from team members about how productive and satisfying they feel the meetings to be, or by monitoring other aspects, such as attendance rate at meetings, the decisions made at meetings, and the number of decisions that result in action.

Further examples of tools that could be used by a practice to build team work and to audit its effectiveness are contained in a distance learning pack (Munro 1991).

TEAMWORK AND QUALITY

Earlier we described how a practice can create teams or working groups to manage particular aspects of their services and the way that the prerequisite for this process was the practice identifying its priorities and specifying areas of work requiring a team approach. Increasingly, one of the main priorities for a practice is the quality of the services that they are providing. This can be seen as a separate managerial or even external activity comparable to the role of the inspector at the end of the production line, or it can become an integral part of every member of the team's daily activity. This approach of total quality management can be implemented in practice in a number of ways. One is to revise the management structure of the practice (Irvine 1990) so that partners have areas of responsibility for which they are accountable, and set clear objectives for these areas to audit their effectiveness. A second approach is to create a quality improvement team brought together specifically to monitor poor quality and solve particular problems.

A third model described earlier is to have working groups within a practice responsible for particular services. They can set targets both for their own work and for the services that are provided. These groups can meet regularly to identify, analyse, and solve problems in order to recommend solutions, in other words, a type of continuous audit constantly striving to enhance quality. It is when these groups are not working effectively, or when the larger team is unhappy about aspects of its performance that the team building and auditing of teamwork itself is required.

CONCLUSION

The fundamental issue in applying audit to teamwork or considering audit by the team is the crucial importance of team involvement and responsibility. A team that does not meet regularly, react honestly with each other, communicate fully, openly and effectively, and in which team members do not learn from each other, cannot function effectively. Teamwork, including audit, requires team time, but wisely invested it should produce considerable returns for the practice.

REFERENCES

Adair, K. (1986). *Effective teambuilding*. Gower, London.
Belbin, R. M. (1981). *Management teams: why they succeed or fail*. Heinemann, London.
Irvine, D. H. (1990). *Managing for quality in general practice*. King's Fund Centre, London.
Munro, K. (1991). *Teamworking in practice: a distance learning package*. Radcliffe Medical Press, Oxford.

APPENDIX

Values checklist — teams and teamwork

1. Work through the following lists of statements and write answers to the questions as quickly as possible. Try to react and write down the first thoughts that occur to you. Values tend to be well established and do not usually require reflective analysis.
2. For this exercise to be useful you must be scrupulously honest with yourself.
3. The statements relate to some key themes/concepts of teamwork.

Take your completed form into the team-based session for discussion with team colleagues.

Equality

1. Should all team members be treated equally?
2. Should all team members be expected to contribute equally to the team task, and to meeting the needs of the team?

Information and power

1. Should all information relevant to the team purpose be shared within the team?
2. How is information shared in your team?
3. Should power be shared by all members of the team? That is:
   (a) The power to take decisions.
   (b) The power to action decisions.
   (c) The power to block decisions.
   (d) The power to commit the team to tasks without consultation.

Team objectives

1. Do you need team objectives if all team members have individual professional objectives?
2. Do you favour compromise in agreeing team objectives?
3. What are the objectives of your team?

Authority

1. Should it be respected?
2. Should it be challenged?

Winning/losing

1. Do you want to win?
2. What does winning mean to you?
3. Do others always have to lose for you to win?
4. What is the attitude towards winning and losing in your team?

Trust

1. What do you mean by trust?
2. How easy do you find it to trust others at work?
3. How easy do you find it to trust others in your team?

Risk taking

1. How comfortable are you with taking risks?
2. What is the attitude in your team towards taking risks?
3. What has influenced this attitude?

Decisions

1. How should teams set about taking decisions?
2. What happens in your team?

Professional standing

1. How much do you respect expertise?
2. How far do academic qualifications affect your valuation of a person's worth?

Openness

1. How far should you carry being truthful?
2. Is it helpful to expose your weaknesses to other members of your team?

Team member characteristics

1. What characteristics are necessary for a person to be a good team member?
2. Are there any characteristics that would render somebody totally unsuitable as a team member?

Leadership

1. Does an effective team require a good leader?
2. What are the qualities of a good leader?
3. How much control should the team leader exert in the team?
4. What kind of leadership style do you think would be most appropriate for your team?
5. Who is your team leader?

18 The primary/secondary care interface

Angela Coulter

CHOOSING THE TOPIC

It is now well established that general practitioners' referral rates often vary widely: studies have demonstrated three- to four-fold variations between practices in the rate at which they refer patients to out-patient clinics, with individual general practitioners' rates being even more variable (Wilkin and Dornan 1990). These variations are indicative of a lack of consensus about the appropriate use of specialist services. For this reason, many general practitioners have been interested in reviewing their performance in this important area, with a view to developing guidelines for referral. As we shall see, this task is far from straightforward.

Referral rates

A common starting point for auditing the interface between primary and secondary care is to collect data on referral rates. All practices are now required to include data on their hospital referrals in their annual reports. The figures have to be broken down by specialty and by hospital, but there is no requirement to present the numbers for individual general practitioners unless practices choose to do it this way. There are considerable difficulties in calculating referral rates for individual general practitioners, as opposed to total rates for the partnership, and it is probably wise not to do so for the purposes of the annual report. However, general practitioners are often keen to compare their own referral patterns with those of their colleagues, so this may be useful for stimulating interest at the start of the audit process.

It is important to remember, however, that referral rates in themselves do not reveal anything very useful about the quality of care. Many studies have attempted to explain the wide differences in referral rates in relation to differential health needs in the practice populations, differences in the availability of hospital services, and differences in the experience and expertise of general practitioners (Wilkin and Smith 1987). None of these factors appear to account for much of the variation and none of them provide any pointers to what a desirable rate of referral would be.

There is no sound reason for believing that the average referral rate is superior to those at either end of the spectrum. High referrers may be accused of generating excessive costs, but doctors with average or low rates may be guilty of withholding beneficial treatment from their patients, possibly resulting in increased costs later on. It is probable that most general practitioners have, on occasions, either referred patients unnecessarily or failed to refer patients who would have benefited from seeing a specialist. This is not surprising, because the referral decision involves assessing a complex array of factors, often in the face of incomplete information about the likely outcome of various options. The aim of reviewing performance in this area is to help general practitioners to improve their ability to make appropriate decisions.

Referral outcomes

In the absence of a consensus about the most desirable rate of referral, it is important that audit groups progress beyond simply comparing rates. Indeed, it could be argued that a focus on rates alone is harmful. An approach which is aimed at identifying and penalizing the outliers (those with high or low rates) runs the risk of alienating them and encouraging complacency in the majority. An educationally sounder approach aims to raise the level of critical awareness more generally. If this is to be achieved, it will be necessary to look at the results or outcomes of referral decisions, with the aim of searching for ways in which the process could be improved to benefit patient care.

The major implication of the research into referral patterns is that the likelihood of referral to a specialist is influenced by factors as yet unidentified, which may be quite distinct from the patient's presenting problem. In other words, faced with the same patient, different doctors make different decisions about the need for specialist intervention.

DEVELOPING GUIDELINES

In common with audits in any other area, an important component of the audit cycle for out-patient referrals is the development of guidelines to assist referral decision-making, incorporating criteria against which performance can be measured. Guidelines can cover general areas concerned with the referral process, for example, topics to be included in referral and discharge letters, information to be given to patients, waiting times, etc., or they can cover topics specific to particular diseases or conditions. The former are much easier to devise than the latter.

General practitioners' reasons for referring patients to out-patient departments divide broadly into three groups: for investigation and diagnosis; for advice and reassurance; for treatment. Any assessment of the appropriateness of referral needs to take account of these different objectives and to try to assess whether the referral was: (a) necessary for this particular patient; (b) timely (neither too early nor too late); and (c) effective (the objectives of the referral were achieved).

Studies have shown that specialists, general practitioners, and patients frequently disagree about when a referral is appropriate (Grace and Armstrong 1986, 1987). There is often disagreement within these groups as well: even specialists working in the same hospital may disagree on quite fundamental aspects of clinical policy. Ideally, guidelines should be based on scientific evidence derived from randomized controlled trials.

The best way of achieving a consensus between all parties is to establish joint working groups between general practitioners and specialists, with sufficient resources to undertake comprehensive reviews of the relevant literature, perhaps supplemented by questionnaire surveys to discover the range of views and practices. These working groups should be locally-based, since the available evidence suggests that guidelines are more likely to be followed if the people who are to implement them have been involved in their development (Roland and Coulter 1992).

COLLECTING THE DATA: REFERRAL RATES

The comparison of referral rates is often quite a good way of starting the audit process, because general practitioners are usually interested to see how their referral patterns compare with others. If a number of practices are involved, they could start by comparing practice-based rates derived from the information in annual reports (Coulter *et al.* 1991*c*).

When comparing practices it is sensible to use the total number of patients on the practice list as the denominator for calculating the rates. It may be appropriate to compare rates for specific age-groups if the age-structures of the practice populations are significantly different.

If those conducting the audit want to calculate referral rates for individual doctors, it will be necessary to use a different denominator. The list size of an individual general practitioner may be a very poor indicator of his or her work-load. It would be better to use number of consultations as the denominator and even better if this included information about the types of clinical problems seen. For example, it is common for a female general practitioner to see many of the patients consulting for gynaecological problems. She is therefore likely to have a higher rate of referral to gynaecology out-patient clinics than her male colleagues, but the reason for the discrepancy will not be clear unless one is able to compare the differences in underlying rates of consultation for these conditions.

It is also important to ensure that the practices whose rates you are comparing have been counting the same things. The following issues need to be considered.

Private referrals

The proportion of patients referred to private clinics can vary considerably from practice to practice and between individual general practitioners. It makes sense to include private referrals in an audit.

Specialty groups

It is usual to group sub-specialties under general specialty headings when studying referrals. It is important to agree on standardized groupings if practice referral rates to individual specialties are to be compared. For example, gastroenterology, cardiology, thoracic medicine, palliative medicine, infectious diseases, and nephrology might all be grouped together with general medicine; while urology could be grouped with general surgery. Numbers referred to some sub-specialties will be too small to make meaningful comparisons between practices, and this will be a frequent problem if one is trying to compare rates for individual doctors (Moore and Roland 1989; Roland *et al.* 1990).

Paramedical referrals

Any comparison of referral rates needs to be clear about whether or not referral to paramedical services is included in the data collection. In some districts general practitioners can refer direct to community psychiatric nurses, whereas in others the initial referral has to be to a consultant psychiatrist. Similarly, some practices have direct access to hearing aid clinics, while others have to refer via ear, nose, and throat consultants. Since the need for hearing aids is a common reason for referring elderly people, direct access to a hearing aid clinic could make a considerable difference to a practice's ear, nose, and throat referral rate.

Referrals by other team members

In certain cases health visitors and other attached staff may have the right to refer patients to hospital services. For the purposes of comparison it will be important to be clear about whether these have been included or excluded.

Self-referrals

Practices often have no means of knowing when their patients are attending accident and emergency departments. However, after the event the practice should receive a hospital discharge note. These could be collated for audit purposes.

In-patient admissions

Hospitals collect data on all admissions, including the name of the patient's general practitioner and practice, so it should be possible to obtain details of numbers of in-patient stays, diagnoses, procedures, length of stay, type of admission, etc. from the district health authority information systems.

EVALUATING THE DATA: REFERRAL RATES

Most studies of referral rates reveal wide variations between practices or between individual general practitioners. This usually stimulates interest in trying to explain the differences. There are a number of possible explanations which should be considered.

Inclusions/exclusions

As mentioned above, it is important to check that the data are comparable. The possibility that some practices have failed to collect complete data should also be considered.

Population differences

A practice that has a large number of elderly people on its list is likely to refer more patients than one with a predominately young population.

Case-mix differences

A practice in a deprived area might be expected to encounter more illness in its population and therefore may have greater need to refer than one in an advantaged area.

Random variation

It is important to be wary of drawing conclusions on the basis of small numbers of referrals. The 95 per cent confidence limits can be quite wide. For example, in a specialty in which the average referral rate is 25 per 1000 patients per year, a practice of 2000 patients would expect a variation of 7 referrals per 1000 patients. In other words, referrals could range from 36 to 64 patients entirely by chance (see pp. 71–2).

Access

As was pointed out above, the availability of various paramedical services may affect referral rates to particular specialties.

If none of the above-mentioned factors can account for the differences, it is reasonable to conclude that the variations are due to differences in practice styles; i.e. general practitioners' decision-making procedures and patterns of care. It then becomes important to try to evaluate these to determine the most appropriate use of specialist services.

COLLECTING AND EVALUATING DATA ON
REFERRAL PROCESS AND OUTCOMES

Case studies of outcomes

Audit groups could select particular 'tracer' conditions (i.e. conditions which are common and interesting for some reason) and examine the case notes of a number of patients who were referred for these problems to see what happened to them. Outcomes to be measured in such a study could include the immediate results of the referral, i.e. the actions initiated by the specialists, and/or longer-term outcomes, such as symptom-prevalence after a specified period of time.

We examined the outcomes of referrals for five common problems (back pain, menstrual disorders, otitis media, deafness, and varicose veins) by conducting a case-note analysis in 20 practices (Coulter *et al.* 1991*a*, *b*). We were able to compare the diagnoses of the general practitioner and the specialist, the tests and investigations ordered by the general practitioner and the specialist, and the treatments initiated by general practitioner and specialist. Data was also obtained on patients' consultations with their general practitioner in the 12 months prior to the index referral, the 12 months after the out-patient appointment, and in the 12 months prior to the case-note study, which took place five years after the index referral. This gave an indication of the extent to which patients were still suffering from the problems for which they were referred.

The problem with this type of study is that it is very difficult to extract reliable data from patients' notes about the relative severity of their condition. Also, the notes rarely include information about the patients' subjective experiences of illness and outcomes and their treatment preferences. Since these are crucial factors in the referral decision, a case-note analysis can only provide a very partial view of the factors influencing outcome.

Studies of referral process

Audit groups might prefer to concentrate on monitoring the referral process, with a view to improving the organizational aspects. The following issues could be considered:

Waiting times

Time from referral to appointment could be measured for particular specialty clinics where a problem is suspected. Results could be discussed with hospital consultants and managers, with the aim of agreeing a strategy for improvement and a target average waiting time plus upper limit. Re-measurement could assess the extent to which the target has been reached.

Attendance rates

The numbers of patients failing to attend out-patient appointments could be counted and the reasons for non-attendance ascertained by means of questionnaires to patients. Agreed changes to appointment systems could be implemented and subsequent attendance rates monitored.

Follow-up consultations

These could be monitored for particular conditions and discussed with hospital staff. Protocols for discharging patients back to general practice care could be agreed and monitored.

Re-referrals and cross referrals

The number of times that patients are re-referred to out-patient clinics or cross-referred from one specialty to another and the reasons for these referrals could be monitored, with the aim of securing improvements in the initial choice of specialist.

Clarification of objectives

General practitioners could record their reasons for referral and assess the results in the light of their expectations. Patients' expectations could be ascertained and included in referral letters.

Communications

Referral and discharge letters could be scrutinized with a view to improving communications. It will be important to consider the amount and breadth of information required, as well as the clarity and timeliness of the communications.

Patient satisfaction

General practitioners might consider organizing surveys of their patients to determine their views of the outpatient services, including such issues as in-clinic waiting times, appointment arrangements, quality, and readability of the information provided, or attitudes of staff. These surveys could be planned in conjunction with community health councils or FHSAs.

IMPLEMENTING CHANGE

Any audit of referrals is likely to throw up a number of ideas for improving the efficiency of the process or for reviewing guidelines. Since this is an area which spans primary and secondary care, it will be necessary to involve clinical and possibly managerial staff in each setting if effective change is to be achieved.

The following examples, taken from our case-note study of the outcomes of referrals, illustrate some of the issues which may arise.

Appropriate access arrangements?

Of the 280 patients referred to ear, nose, and throat departments for deafness, 45 per cent received only a hearing aid. This involved a cross-referral to the hearing aid technician, with another appointment and another long wait for the patient. This raises the question of whether it is necessary to insist that these patients see an ear, nose, and throat specialist, or whether general practitioners should be free to refer them directly to hearing aid technicians.

Appropriate referral?

Of the 182 patients referred for back pain, 46 per cent had been referred before, with 9 per cent having had more than 5 previous referrals. Since there is very little evidence that any treatments for back pain are effective, the fact that there are multiple referrals for this condition suggests that there may be scope for rationalizing the process. Some people have argued that patients with chronic low back problems could be more thoroughly assessed in specialist back pain clinics where they could see a range of specialist and paramedical staff and where they could be given advice on how to manage their condition and prevent recurrence.

Appropriate investigation?

Of the 145 patients referred for menorrhagia, half underwent dilatation and curettage including 40 per cent of those aged under 35. This is surprising, because the scientific literature would suggest that this procedure has no therapeutic effect and its value as a diagnostic tool in women in the younger age-group is doubtful, to say the least. This is a clear case for developing guidelines for referral, involving both general practitioners and gynaecologists in a careful review of the scientific evidence on which policy should be based.

Appropriate follow-up arrangements?

Of the 89 children who had grommets inserted following referral for otitis media, 55 per cent had two or more follow-up appointments in the out-patient department and many were kept under specialist care for a considerable period of time, probably at some inconvenience to the patients and their parents. This raised the question of whether general practitioners could take over responsibility for routine follow-up. Following discussion between consultants and general practitioners at a local level and the provision of training and information, a general practitioner follow-up system has been implemented.

REPEATING THE AUDIT

There is a dearth of published examples of general practice audits of referrals which have completed the cycle and achieved change. However, the following three examples cover the primary/secondary care interface and, although they were not initiated by general practitioners, they may provide useful models for general practice audit groups.

The first example is an audit initiated by a group of consultant physicians in a teaching hospital in Wales who were concerned about the number of follow-up appointments in their general medicine out-patient clinics (Hall *et al.* 1988). Details of all new out-patients referred to the clinics of eight consultants and their junior staff were monitored on a simple form. Guidelines were then drawn up and issued to four of the eight clinics. The guidelines covered the following issues:

1. New patients should normally be seen once only and discharged to the care of the referring doctor.
2. A follow-up appointment should only be given if there is (a) diagnostic uncertainty requiring further assessment; (b) need to monitor a complex disease; and (c) serious disease requiring further investigation and treatment by a specialist rather than a general practitioner.
3. A further appointment should not be made simply to give the patient the results of tests.
4. Diagnostic tests should only be used if the results will alter a decision.
5. Referring doctors should normally be sent information, including the results of tests, within ten days of the out-patient appointment or in-patient discharge.

At the end of the nine month study, the four 'guideline' clinics were found to have discharged 47 per cent of patients, as against 28 per cent in the control clinics, and the mean number of diagnostic tests had been reduced to 1 per patient, as against 2 in the control group. The ratio of total to new attenders had been reduced to 3:1 in the guideline clinics, compared with 7.8:1 for Wales as a whole. The authors argue that if the higher rate of discharge was to be achieved by all consultant general physicians in Wales, the general medical out-patient waiting list would be eliminated in three to six months.

The second example was the result of an initiative by public health physicians in the Northern Regional Health Authority (Donaldson and Hill 1991). Concerned about patterns of use of the domiciliary consultation service, they audited its use by extracting data from claim forms and by prospective data collection. This revealed large variations in styles of practice and many departures from the criteria on which eligibility to perform the service is based: in particular, the requirement that the general practitioner accompany the consultant was met in only 1 out of every 17 cases.

The result of this exercise was that use of the domiciliary consultation service declined in the Northern region by 53 per cent over four years, which was considerably in excess of the national rate of decline of 27 per cent. Savings of £604 000 were achieved and the authors concluded that the peer review exercise had proved effective in rationalizing use of the service.

The third example was the result of a collaboration between rheumatologists, public health physicians, and general practitioners in Guy's Hospital, London (Grahame *et al.* 1986). Their starting point was the desire to encourage general practitioners to undertake more diagnosis and treatment of common rheumatic conditions, so as to spare patients the inconvenience and delay in seeking hospital advice.

They initiated a training programme for general practitioners which included instruction on (a) practical advice on the precise diagnosis of common lesions; (b) the indications for local steroid injections and supervised practice of injection techniques for painful shoulder, epicondylitis, carpal tunnel syndrome, etc.; (c) the use and abuse of anti-rheumatic drugs; and (d) the optimal use of physiotherapy and occupational therapy services in rheumatic disorders.

All patients with fresh episodes of upper-limb pain consulting their general practitioners over a 3-month period before and after were indexed and their precise diagnoses, treatment, and progress were charted by a research assistant. The authors reported a number of improvements in the care of patients following the training programme: there was an increase in use of corticosteroid injections; a reduction in the use of non-steroidal drugs for arm-pain conditions; a reduced use of investigations and referrals; and an increase in the proportion of patients treated 'appropriately' (as judged by the consultants) from 43 per cent to 66 per cent.

The published papers do not indicate whether the authors went on to repeat the audit cycle to see if these improvements were maintained, nor whether or not the guidelines were reassessed. Nevertheless, they provide a useful model of how the audit process can achieve measurable improvements, at least in the short term.

CONCLUSION

The audit of referrals is one of the more difficult areas in which to produce valid data and demonstrate change. Nevertheless, it is an increasingly important topic as primary and secondary care become more integrated and there is a chance to show that well-conducted audit in this area does stimulate change.

REFERENCES

Coulter, A., Bradlow, J., Agass, M., Martin-Bates, C., and Tulloch, A. (1991*a*). Outcomes of referrals for menstrual problems: an audit of general practice records. *Journal of the Royal College of Obstetrics and Gynaecology*, **98**, 789–96.

Coulter, A., Bradlow, J., Martin-Bates, C., Agass, M., and Tulloch, A. (1991*b*). Outcome of general practitioner referrals to specialist outpatient clinics for back pain. *British Journal of General Practice*, **41**, 450–3.

Coulter, A., Roland, M., and Wilkin, D. (1991*c*). *GP referrals to hospital*. Centre for Primary Care Research, Manchester.

Donaldson, L. and Hill, P. (1991). The domiciliary consultation service: time to take stock. *British Medical Journal*, **302**, 449–51.

Grace, J. F. and Armstrong, D. (1986). Reasons for referral to hospital: extent of agreement between the perceptions of patients, general practitioners and consultants. *Family Practice*, **3**, 143–7.

Grace, J. F. and Armstrong, D. (1987). Referral to hospital: perceptions of patients, general practitioners and consultants about necessity and suitability of referral. *Family Practice*, **4**, 170–5.

Grahame, R., Gibson, T., Dale, E., Anderson, J., Brown, R., Higgins, P., and Curwen, M. (1986). An evaluated programme of rheumatology training for general practitioners. *British Journal of Rheumatology*, **25**, 7–12.

Hall, R., Roberts, C., Coles, G., Fisher, D., Fowkes, F., Jones, J. *et al.* (1988). The impact of guidelines in clinical outpatient practice. *Journal of the Royal College of Physicians of London*, **22**, 244–7.

Moore, A. T. and Roland, M. O. (1989). How much variation in referral rates among general practitioners is due to change? *British Medical Journal*, **298**, 500–502.

Roland, M. O. and Coulter, A. (1992). *Hospital referrals*. Oxford University Press.

Roland, M. O., Bartholomew, J., Morrell, D. C., McDermott, A., and Paul, E. (1990). Understanding hospital referral rates: a users' guide. *British Medical Journal*, **301**, 98–102.

Wilkin, D. and Dornan, C. (1990). *General practitioner referrals to hospital: a review of research and its implications for policy and practice*. Centre for Primary Care Research, Manchester.

Wilkin, D. and Smith, A. (1987). Explaining variation in general practitioner referrals to hospital. *Family Practice*, **4**, 160–9.

19   Practice visiting

Theo Schofield

Earlier chapters in this book have described methods of auditing particular aspects of a practice and its work. This chapter will consider methods that can be used to make more global evaluations of the whole practice by visiting. The methodology was originally designed by a working party of the Royal College of General Practitioners, and described in their report 'What sort of doctor?' (1981). It has since been developed for assessing training practices and for practice team visiting.

WHAT SORT OF DOCTOR?

The remit of the first 'What sort of doctor?' working party was to devise a method for established general practitioners to evaluate their performance in the setting of their own practices. It was seen as an educational method which would enable doctors to receive feedback about the strengths and weaknesses of their own practice and to encourage continued development, but the potential for assessment for Fellowship or Membership of the College or for re-accreditation was also recognized.

CHOOSING THE TOPIC

The four areas of performance that the working party selected were:

1. Professional values—the doctor's perception of his or her role in relation to individual patients and the practice community; ideals and sense of priorities; the spirit which motivates and guides the gradual evolution of the practice.
2. Clinical competence—the technical aspects of the doctor's work, commonly understood as medical.
3. Accessibility—the ease with which the community of patients have access to the practice and to the facilities within it. The doctor's own availability.
4. Ability to communicate—ability to get on the same wavelength as the patients whatever their background. Receptiveness and ability to convey thoughts accurately to practice staff and colleagues within the practice and outside.

Though there was some overlap between these areas the working party would demonstrate that they were capable of separate evaluation.

AGREEING CRITERIA

The first task was to define the essential attributes that a doctor needed to be an effective practitioner in each of these areas. For example, the first criterion of professional values was 'that the doctor sees himself as providing a service to his practice population, sharing with others the responsibility for promoting, preserving, and restoring the health of individual patients'. The opposite of this was 'the doctor regarding medical practice solely as a way of earning a living while encountering interesting clinical material'. Similar criteria were drawn up in each of the four areas, 35 in all.

The working party did not attempt to define a level of performance for each criterion which could be considered acceptable, partly because one aim was to encourage movement rather than to make pass or fail judgements, and partly because allowance needed to be made for local circumstances when assessing the degree of achievement of an individual doctor.

SOURCES OF INFORMATION

The method of assessment was based on a visit to the doctor's own practice by two of his colleagues for the best part of the day. The assessment had six components.

1. Study of the practice profile which comprised a completed questionnaire circulated to the assessors in advance of the visit recording the salient features of the practice.
2. Direct observation of the practice premises, its facilities and equipment and the way it functioned.
3. Discussion with ancillary staff and other members of the practice's health care team.
4. Inspection of individual clinical records and any registers or indexes the practice possessed.
5. Review of a videotape of a series of the doctor's recent consultations together with the relevant records.
6. An interview with the doctor to elicit his or her views and understanding on a variety of topics, including material derived from randomly selected records of patients.

The advantages of this method were that the assessment was based on direct observation of the doctor's performance in practice and that each method of assessment provided information from which performance in a number of areas could be assessed.

Apart from the time-consuming nature of this evaluation, difficulties included identifying the individual doctor's contribution to the way that the practice ran as a whole, and having fairly limited information on which to base the assessment of clinical competence.

EVALUATING THE DATA

Doctors in practices who have been involved in this sort of assessment visit almost universally comment on how much they have learnt from the opportunity of visiting other practices as well as having their own work assessed. At the end of the visit the visitors produce a written report summarizing the strengths and weaknesses that they have identified in each of the four areas of performance. The more the comments are specifically related to the criteria and based on specific information gained during the visit, and the more that these observations are coupled to specific recommendations for change, the greater the value of the report to the doctor and to practice which is being visited.

During the initial pilot trials of this form of visiting many practices commented that the report crystallized a number of things of which they were aware already but that the assessment encouraged them to confront these issues. Some reported quite major changes as a result of their visit (Royal College of General Practitioners 1985).

CONCLUSION

Avedis Donabedian visited the UK in 1984 and took part in a number of 'What sort of doctor?' visits. He later wrote

I'm impressed, challenged and deeply moved by it. I find it admirable in concept and overall design, and as a method of assessment. As to its conceptual foundations and overall design, this is a formulation unique, as far as I know, in the range, depth, and richness of what it perceives the quality of care to be; and particularly so in its recognition that values are the source from which every other virtue must necessarily flow. And there is more. 'What sort of doctor?' recognizes the interrelationship of the organizational features of a practice and the practitioners' performance. It shows awareness of the interdependence of general practitioners, other health care professionals, and supporting staff. It builds directly on the only firm foundation for professional excellence: the sharing of knowledge between peers, the assumption of personal responsibility by individual practitioners, and the commitment to a lifetime of learning through continual self-study.

The proposals offered by 'What sort of doctor?' are also admirable in many ways as a method of assessment. They demonstrate a commitment to measuring, even if imperfectly, that which is truly important rather than only that which can be precisely measured. They envisage a synthesis of mutually supportive or mutually corrective information of several kinds from a variety of sources, videotaping being only the most novel and arresting. The method proposed is also characterized by a delicate balancing of directiveness and flexibility: while principles, objectives, and criteria are unequivocally declared, the standards of performance that may reasonably be attained are subject to local adjustment through negotiation among peers.

(Donabedian 1986)

With such a ringing endorsement, why has this method of mutual evaluation not been universally adopted? There are undoubtedly some reservations about the design, some of which, for example the difficulty of assessing clinical competence and identifying the contribution of individual practitioners, have already been mentioned. Practice visiting does not easily fit in to the established pattern of continued medical education and is relatively time-consuming, even though three days spent practice visiting may be of much greater value than a three day refresher course.

Perhaps the most powerful block has been a reluctance of doctors to expose themselves to such close scrutiny and an understandable reluctance on the part of visitors to assess and make judgements about their colleagues. This last problem can largely be overcome by training and experience which enables visitors to make more reliable judgements and to comment in ways that are acceptable and constructive.

'What sort of doctor?' has the essential strength of review by peers who share the same perspective and problems as the doctor they are assessing. It is also a powerful tool for evaluation and for change and Medical Audit Advisory Groups in particular might look at it afresh to consider whether it is a professional activity that they wish to develop.

APPROVAL OF TRAINERS IN TRAINING PRACTICES

An alternative way in which practice visiting could develop is illustrated by the mechanisms of approval of trainers and training practices which have been developed in the Oxford Regional Vocational Training Scheme. In this instance there is a defined service that a practice can apply to provide—teaching a trainee; a regulatory body with responsibility for ensuring that the service is delivered and that the consumer's needs are met; and a contract which has to be renewed every four years. It does not take too much imagination to envisage the ways in which this scenario could be applied to other services and other contracts, and this could be a very positive or an extremely damaging development. Based on the experience of vocational training schemes over the past 10 years it is possible to describe a number of essential requirements that will ensure that assessment visiting for the purpose of performance review is valuable (Schofield and Hasler 1984).

1. *The criteria used for the assessment should be based on the consumers' needs.* In the case of the training practices a statement of principle was made

that 'Teaching practices and trainers are selected for the educational opportunities they offer their trainees. Since trainees may learn from the experience and example of working in the practice as well as from teaching and other educational resources, all these areas must be examined.

2. *The criteria must be agreed by those who are to be assessed.* This may involve a fairly lengthy period of consultation, and some of the methods that have been used to agree criteria have been discussed in an earlier chapter in this book.

3. *The criteria must be realistic, and acceptable levels of performance must be defined in relation to local circumstances.* At one extreme one must avoid setting unattainable ideals and at the other failing to meet the responsibilities to the consumer by making too much allowance for the problems of the practice.

4. *All practitioners should be involved as assessors.* This gives all practitioners the opportunity to learn from visiting each other's practices, but more importantly creates a sense of involvement in the whole process. It avoids a 'them and us' feeling and is another safeguard to ensure that the judgements that are made are realistic.

5. *Assessors must receive training.* Teams of two or three general practitioners are led by an experienced visitor who has the responsibility for conducting the visit and writing the report.

6. *The report should be based on informed judgements against the agreed criteria.* The report should make clear what information has been gathered in the practice and the degree to which individual criteria have or have not been met. General statements, such as 'The practice has a nice atmosphere', are far less valuable than noting that 'The practice has regular meetings and all members of staff are able to add items to the agenda and feel able to express their ideas freely'. Another dimension of experience is to be able to make recommendations, based not just on one's own practice, but also on ideas from other practices that have been visited.

7. *The ethos of the assessment should be to encourage development.* The purpose of assessment visiting should be to develop the services that the practices are providing. The final report of the process should identify areas in which the practice should be encouraged to develop and practices should expect to improve levels of performance between one evaluation and the next. It is also possible over time for the criteria and the acceptable levels of performance to increase as the overall standard of the practices develops.

8. *Resources should be available to encourage practice development.* There is little point in identifying the areas of weakness if the means of improving them are not available. In the context of training, this means the provision of teachers' courses, courses on teaching of communication skills, practice management, etc., but if this method was applied in other settings education provision would again need to be made for teams to develop the necessary skills to meet the criteria.

Vocational training is just one example of a situation in which there is a fine balance to be maintained between centrally determined targets, local contracting and management, and individual practice responsibility. It is also an example of a situation in which the profession has retained the responsibility for maintaining standards and has not shied away from some difficult decisions in individual cases. It may be that the profession needs to consider whether it wishes to take the same route in other areas.

PRACTICE TEAM VISITING

A development of the 'What sort of doctor?' approach has been to expand the focus of the evaluation from the individual doctor to the practice team, involving a multi-disciplinary team in the assessment with the aim of enabling practices to help each other to improve their preventive care, chronic disease management, and health promotion (ACT 1990).

Visits are arranged between pairs of practices, who visit each other in turn. The visiting team includes as a core a general practitioner, a practice nurse, and a practice manager but may also include a district nurse, health visitor, and other reception or clerical staff. The team assess the structure of the practice's arrangements for managing preventive care and chronic disease and its involvement in health promotion, and the process of care as demonstrated by audits already conducted by the practice. The evaluation is based on analysis of a practice profile or report, together with structured interviews between team members. After the visit a report is written which emphasizes the practice strengths and includes constructive suggestions for improvements.

An added benefit of this style of visitng is the extent to which it brings the team together both as visitors to plan their assessment and as the home team to consider how they are going to present their work.

CONCLUSION

Direct observation and evaluation of one's work by one's peers is probably the most penetrating, and therefore a very valuable although threatening, form of performance review. It takes time to agree the criteria and prepare the visits, to conduct the visits themselves, and to write a report and respond to its conclusions. The methodology has not been subjected to a rigorous evaluation, but doctors and practice teams which have been involved have consistently reported how much they have learnt both about their own practice and from those that they have visited, and a remarkable degree of change has been stimulated as a result. There is therefore a strong case for considering and developing this methodology further.

REFERENCES

ACT. (1990). *Practice team visiting* (ed. M. S. Lawrence and M. Tettersall). ACT, Oxford.

Donabedian, A. (1986). Impression of a journey in Britain. In *In pursuit of quality* (ed. D. Pendleton, T. Schofield and M. Marinker). Royal College of General Practitioners, London.

Royal College of General Practitioners. (1981). What sort of doctor? *Journal of the Royal College of General Practitioners*, **31**, 698–702.

Royal College of General Practitioners. (1985). What sort of doctor? *Assessing quality of care in general practice. Report from general practice 23*. RCGP, London.

Schofield, T. P. C. and Hasler, J. C. (1984). Approved of trainers and training practices in the Oxford Region. *British Medical Journal*, **288**, 538–40, 612–14, 688–9.

Part IV
Support and evaluation

20 The role of the Medical Audit Advisory Group

Alan Forbes and Martin Lawrence

BACKGROUND

In 1987 the Government began changes to the NHS with a White Paper entitled 'Promoting better health' (Secretaries of State 1987). A second White Paper, 'Working for patients', was followed by the imposition of a new general practitioner contract, and relations between the profession and government became very hostile, with general practitioners angry, distrustful, and dispirited (Secretaries of State 1989; Department of Health 1989).

Yet within this legislation were proposals for the enhancement of audit in the health service in general and in primary care in particular. Even opponents of the new contract usually agree that this initiative offered great opportunity for the profession, but even this benefit may be lost unless the opportunity is taken up.

Working Paper 6 of 'Working for patients' was on the subject of audit and stated clearly that 'the Goverment's approach is based firmly on the principle that the quality of medical work can only be reviewed by a doctor's peers' but it went on to make a rather political definition of audit 'the systematic, critical analysis of medical care, including the procedures used for diagnosis and treatment, the use of resources, and the resulting outcome and quality of life for the patient'; it referred to only one example, which was of 'external audit by peers in general practice'; it stated that 'where necessary management must be able to institute an independent audit. This may take the form of external peer review or joint professional and management appraisal'; and it stated that 'the general practitioners' terms of service will be amended to include a requirement to participate in medical audit'. The envisaged management role in audit was clear, but later developments have emphasized the potential for the exercise to be professionally led.

FACILITIES FOR MEDICAL AUDIT ADVISORY GROUPS (MAAGs)

The crucial document for audit in primary health care is government circular HC(FP) (90)8, a poorly produced circular consisting of a single, folded A4 sheet, but containing some important and beneficial directives for primary care audit (Department of Health 1990). It instructs each FHSA to set up a MAAG to 'direct, co-ordinate, and monitor medical audit activities in all general medical practices in the area'. It then continues to make some important statements about how such a group should work.

First, the document states some background principles. 'Audit will be professionally led'. 'An effective programme of audit will give reassurance to patients, doctors and managers' (this implies that the knowledge of the existence of an effective programme should be adequate for public accountability without publication of the detail). 'FHSAs have a responsibility to oversee the quality of service provided. (They) will need mechanisms independent of the medical audit system, to consider wider issues of quality and ensure contractual obligations are fulfilled.' (This absolves the MAAG from having to perform the function of policeman, and enables it to concentrate on an educational approach.)

Secondly, the document is clear about the need for confidentiality. It states that the MAAG must 'cast reports in such a form that individual patients and doctors cannot be identified'; and with regard to records of problems found through audit it states that 'these records must be regarded as confidential to the MAAG'.

Thirdly, it makes explicit that 'resources have been made available to the FHSA . . . to enable the MAAG and its audit teams to carry out their responsibilities'.

In these short instructions the Government made clear that it intended that FHSAs should set up professional, confidential, and well-resourced audit advisory groups to help practices with medical audit.

OBLIGATIONS OF MAAGs

The MAAG should 'provide the Family Practitioner Committee with the general results of the audit programme'; and it should be accountable for 'the institution of regular and systematic audit in which all practices take part'; and it should 'establish appropriate mechanisms to ensure that problems revealed through audit are solved'.

While there is no difficulty with the first of these obligations, there is clear incompatibility between the other two and the conditions stated above under which MAAGs have been established. Thus, it is not possible to guarantee audit 'in all practices' when this has been removed as a term of service; nor to ensure that all 'problems revealed through audit are solved' in an environment where the identity of the doctor or practice in question may not be revealed.

A CODE OF CONDUCT

For this reason many MAAGs have felt it necessary to publish an explicit Code of Conduct, making it clear to both practices and the FHSA how they intend to walk this tightrope between confidentiality and accountability. For example, at Liverpool it was agreed that:

1. Practices are able to decide on the level of disclosure of information collected by the audit facilitators:
   (a) to the facilitator and no further;
   (b) to the MAAG;
   (c) to the FHSA.
2. No non-aggregated data will ever be disclosed to any third party (including the FHSA) without the consent of all the practitioners concerned on each occasion.
3. Only the MAAG's administrative assistant and the facilitators have access to the data stored on the MAAG's computer.

Such a strict code of confidentiality is clearly necessary if practices are to join with the MAAG in undertaking an honest appraisal of their activities. Without the reassurance of confidentiality, practices cannot be open or honest, and so the educational opportunity would be lost.

Conversely, there remains the need to reassure both patients, Health Authority, and Government that audit is adequate and that the quality of care is being assured. Questions asked of the MAAG include 'What will you do if audit reveals inadequate medical care, or even dangerous practice?', or 'What will you do if you find that a practice is providing false evidence to the FHSA to obtain resources?'. This certainly is a major problem, because on the one hand a MAAG is obliged to 'Deal with problems revealed by audit' but, on the other hand, is bound to maintain confidentiality. MAAGs have overwhelmingly agreed that both the need for confidentiality in order to develop effective medical audit, and the need to conform to the strictures of the Government's health circular, imply that confidentiality should be the overriding factor. In order to clarify the position, both to the FHSA and to practices, some MAAGs have published specific guidelines on what would be done if problems were to be revealed by audit. For instance, the policy of the Oxford MAAG is:

1. Any problem revealed through audit will be managed by means of education only.
2. The audit co-ordinator (facilitator) will offer to discuss the problem with the practice and suggest educational opportunities if appropriate.
3. The MAAG chairperson or other appropriate MAAG member will offer to attend practice to provide advice and help with change.
4. If no improvement occurs, the MAAG will still not reveal confidential information to the FHSA or any third party. It will be bound to report in general terms the number of practices in Oxfordshire which may be inadequate in certain respects (and will point out to the practice the consequent effect on the profession's standing in Oxfordshire).

On this basis the MAAG was able to go forward to develop confidential medical audit, confident that it was both in accordance with the Government's circular, and that it was adequately accountable to patients and the Health Authority.

THE DEVELOPMENT OF A MAAG: THE EXAMPLE OF LIVERPOOL

When the Department of Health funded four pilot projects to run in 1990, the Chairperson and General Manager of the Liverpool FHSA, the Professor of General Practice at Liverpool University and the Secretary of the Liverpool Local Medical Committee decided to bid for funding, and were accepted. A shadow MAAG was formed for 11 months from February through December 1990. It consisted of eight representatives of general practice (appointed by the Local Medical Committee, the Regional Advisor, the RCGP, and the University Department), a hospital consultant (by government instruction), and an officer of the FHSA.

The first decision was that any prescriptive action should be delayed until the state of audit in Liverpool general practice had been ascertained. Early discussions resulted in an explicit statement of aims:

1. To establish the level of audit at the time the MAAG was formed.
2. To encourage audit in all practices.
3. To improve the quality of existing audit, concentrating on clinical rather than managerial aspects.
4. To protect confidentiality.
5. To motivate, stimulate, develop, and foster audit.

These aims are similar to but not identical to those laid down by the Department of Health (Department of Health 1990). From the outset Liverpool FHSA has adopted a management style which indicated that they were comfortable with professional leadership in audit. Any FHSA which sees the audit system in a regulatory way may appear to gain control over audit locally, but such an approach would strangle educational audit. In particular, the management and regulatory role of Independent Medical Advisors to FHSAs makes their regular attendance at MAAG meetings inappropriate.

In order to liaise with practices and to establish the level of audit activity in Liverpool, two recently retired, well-respected, local general practitioners were appointed as audit facilitators. (Other MAAGs have since followed a similar line, but some have appointed younger general practitioners with, for example, two sessions a week; others have appointed non-doctors as facilitators). All the practices within Liverpool were visited within four months. The first contact was by letter, in which the professional nature of the project was emphasized.

These early visits were met with a great deal of suspicion, and the facilitators were asked to explore the situation very tentatively. Answers were sought to the questions: 'What audit is already taking place?', 'What barriers exist?', 'What help is needed to promote audit of high quality?'. It was helpful for the facilitator to meet as many of the practice as were willing, and for the practice to identify a contact person for ease of communication in the future.

Confidentiality

In setting up the structure of the MAAG there was great concern with confidentiality. The only feasible location for the office was in the FHSA building; but the office was quite separate and locked. It has been equipped with a direct telephone line independent of the FHSA switchboard, and has a distinct delivery address with its own Post Office box number.

An administrative assistant was appointed, with skills in several important areas, such as collection, collation, and analysis of complicated data, use of computers and application of meticulous attention to detail.

Information held in the MAAG office has been coded, so only the audit administrator and the facilitators know exactly which individual practices in Liverpool are performing audit in any one clinical area unless the practice has given permission for its name and specific interests to appear in the current audit directory. This now lists a combination of 30 subject areas and 50 practices willing to share ideas.

Members of the MAAG also had to decide on a method of working between the MAAG and the FHSA. In Liverpool it was agreed that an FHSA representative should be on the MAAG, and that meetings should be split into two parts. The first part, attended by all including the FHSA representative, was for management topics, and the second, for which the FHSA member withdrew, was designated 'For confidential items'. In practice, after the first few meetings, there was rarely a need for the FHSA representative to withdraw, but the facility is still formally available should any sensitive issues arise. (Other MAAGs have used different solutions. In Oxfordshire, for instance, there are two committees, the MAAG, which is entirely professional, and the Quality Improvement Group (QUIG) on which both FHSA staff, lay members, and several MAAG members sit. This ensures communication and co-operation while maintaining the independence of the MAAG.)

Working together

Early meetings were characterized by a developing unity. Issues were thoroughly discussed and decisions made by consensus. The FHSA member recalls being very frustrated, but now agrees that a refusal to be rushed paid dividends later. The hospital consultant could not contribute much at that time, other than reassurance that hospital audit was in a similar state of uncertainty;

our experience is that the appointment of this secondary care representative should be delayed for six to twelve months.

The members all worked together. There was no obvious way in which the general practitioners behaved differently according to which body or organizaion they represented. If there were any hidden agendas they were very well hidden. The academic general practitioner contributed without in any way appearing to teach the rest.

Advice was sought from several outsiders, for example a pharmacy adviser and a health promotion facilitator (who continues to attend as an observer). A social scientist with expertise in gathering and interpreting patients' views became part of a patient satisfaction sub-group. A representative from a local Community Health Council made many important suggestions which contrasted starkly with ideas about numerical audit. 'Is it possible to measure attitudes, treating people with dignity, giving patients time to talk, talking to patients in a language they can understand, taking time to listen, providing the patient with as much information as possible about him or herself, encouraging the patient to participate in making choices? Can the 'communicating' role of a doctor be audited?'

Open meeting

The first open meeting, 'Audit—friend or foe?' was an attempt to demystify audit. A total of 104 doctors from 71 practices (out of 110—65 per cent) met. The MAAG introduced itself with two talks—the first 'What MAAG is' and the second 'What MAAG is not'. These talks were much less important than the questions which followed. Members were bombarded with a number of vehement attacks, particularly against academic general practice and the Local Medical Committee's representatives for allowing the Government to 'do these things to us'. Much anxiety and anger was freely expressed, but the airing, and where appropriate answering or acceptance, of criticism allowed subsequent small group work to be constructive. The groups worked on 'What frightens me about audit', and a summary of some of the fears are shown in Table 20.1. The meeting included an analysis of data from the practice visits, showing the factors making audit more or less likely. Practices with trainees, several partners, a practice manager, and a tradition of holding clinical meetings between partners were auditing more than average. Recent acquisition of a computer, involvement in a cost-rent scheme, or changes in practice staff were all quoted as reasons for delaying the start of audit. Single-handedness made audit less likely. The need for a single-handed doctor group had been identified by the facilitators; recruitment began at the open day, its first meeting occurred later that month and it very soon became autonomous.

Helping practices

'Audit—friend or foe?' resulted in a whole range of practical requests (Table 20.2). The MAAG has attempted to provide all of them. Initially members felt

Table 20.1 *Summary of fears expressed in small groups*

1. Lack of knowledge
   (a) What is audit?
   (b) Why do audit?
   (c) Where to start?
2. Fear of imposition
   (a) Who sets the standards?
   (b) Will they be universally applied?
   (c) Will it be done for management and not educational reasons?
   (d) Will doctors only audit easily measurable areas?
3. Fear of consequences
   (a) What will be the outcome?
   (b) Will it improve care?
   (c) Will it lead to cash limiting?
   (d) Will doctors be victims of self-inflicted consequences?
4. Practical fears
   (a) Not enough time.
   (b) Not enough staff.
   (c) Staff not willing/trained.
   (d) How much will it cost?
5. Confidentiality.

Table 20.2 *What general practitioners wanted from MAAG*

1. Dissemination of ideas
2. Protocols for audit
3. Guidance
4. A forum for comparison
5. Resources/information
6. Ideas on areas to be audited
7. Facilitation
8. Meetings between like-minded general practitioners
9. Local audit groups
10. Newsletter/regular communication
11. Arrangements for general practitioners to visit other practices
12. Representation of overseas doctors, female doctors, involvement of practice staff

that off-the-shelf protocols might inhibit true self examination. But it has become clear that many practices benefit from some guidelines in developing their audits.

Local audit groups have had variable impact. Many doctors use their group practice as their local group. Some of the group work includes consideration of contacts with secondary care; for instance, one group has met with a consultant psychiatrist, looked at current psychiatric referrals, and hopes to set and monitor explicit guidelines for such referrals. Much valuable work can take place in groups, and if doctors work within their group practices then it is important that there is some form of cross-fertilizing experience. Considerable effort has been made to promote the involvement of the whole practice team in audit. Educational courses have been run for staff, and the involvement of nurse, practice manager, and reception staff has already increased.

The first newsletter, *MAAGAZINE*, included a questionnaire seeking feedback. Sixty per cent of Liverpool practices responded, and of these 60 per cent said that their attitude to audit had changed because of the facilitators' visit and/or the open day. Specific comments were generally favourable.

Medical students and audit

The newsletter also introduced a fresh initiative from the local department of general practice, which has been supportive throughout. Each academic term, 50 first clinical year medical students have spent one week in practices doing project work planned by the students and the academic department. This year practices were invited to bid for 3–5 students to assist in audit projects. The students were able to select an audit project, do the work, and report back to the academic department and someone from the practice within a week. The students and general practitioners learned much about audit, the students a great deal about general practice, and the practices received a piece of audit work to build on. Table 20.3 shows the range of topics audited in this way.

All but one of the practices involved at the start submitted bids for the second round, and, in the view of the department of general practice, the quality improved the second time.

Outcome

A second open day was held at the end of the pilot year. That day included a series of reports of audit projects, some fostered by the MAAG, and included work by a practice manager, a student, and a trainee. The MAAG had been struck by the vehemence of doctors' response at the first open day. At the second meeting, each of the anxieties expressed six months earlier were recalled and addressed.

All of the Liverpool practices were visited during the year by the facilitators. Table 20.4 summarizes the uptake of MAAG activities. The fact that only 6 of the 105 practices have attended no voluntary meeting encourages belief that the low-key, non-threatening approach has been appropriate.

A very difficult aspect of audit activity to measure is change. Was there any change in attitude towards audit or in audit activity in Liverpool during the year? Soft indicators were an improved atmosphere for the second facilitator visits and the almost complete absence of anger and suspicion at the second open day. A

Table 20.3 *Student audit projects*

Round 1

Patient satisfaction re: appointment system
Cardiovascular risk factors
Prescribing for the elderly
Blood pressure recording/smoking recording/cardiovascular risk factors
Hormone replacement therapy
Epilepsy
Asthma
Minor surgery
Consultation rates

Round 2

Well-woman clinic
Care of the terminally ill
Diabetes clinic
Repeat perscribing
Use of medical services by nursing homes
Evaluation of the consultation
Well-baby clinic
Minor surgery
Depo Provera uptake
Quality of diabetic care

Table 20.4 *Uptake of MAAG activities: Feb–Dec 1990 (105 practices including 40 single-handed practices)*

First open meeting	69 practices
Single-handed doctors' group	27 doctors
Locality based audit groups	33 practices
Student projects	14 practices
Second open meeting	52 practices

81 practices (77 per cent) have taken part in at least one open meeting.
55 practices (52 per cent) have attended at least one meeting of either the Single-handed Doctors Group or a Locality Based Audit Group.

6   practices have not responded to any of the MAAG activities.
2   of these 6 practices were engaged in audit in both March and November.
4   practices are *not* engaged in audit have *not* participaed in any of the MAAG activities.

more firm indicator was that by the second facilitator visits the level of activity had roughly doubled. It is hard to be precise, because the audit facilitators were more strict over what they classed as audit, while the practices were more experienced in claiming activity as audit. However, such a large change has to be encouraging—and data collected after a further year show that the percentage of practices undertaking audit continues to increase (Fig. 20.1).

FUTURE DIRECTIONS FOR MAAG ACTIVITY

The example of Liverpool has been quoted at length because it illustrates well the challenges of establishing audit in an area where many practices are working in adverse conditions, and many are hostile or fearful of audit. It also shows the benefit of working with practices; of helping them to improve their own audit activities rather than imposing from above; and of acknowledging and working with doctors' antagonism. It is notable though, that one of the constant findings in bottom-up assessment is that practices want some top-down help. There are several ways in which the MAAG can work to help practices improve their audits more rigorously and quickly.

Staff support

As well as appointing general practitioner facilitators, many MAAGs are now appointing non-doctor facilitators, with a background of practice nursing, health visitoring, managing, or other primary care roles. The advantage is that these

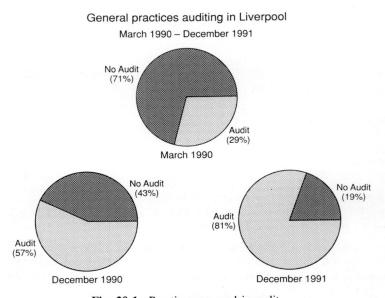

Fig. 20.1 Practices engaged in audit.

professionals may have a closer understanding of some of the activities being audited and for the staff who are increasingly doing audit. Also, MAAGs can afford to employ more hours of non-doctor time. An alternative role for MAAGs is to help practices to bid for more FHSA resources. It must be made clear that this does *not* mean that the MAAG uses confidential audit material to bid on behalf of the practice—but it can help the practice prepare its own bid.

Auditing audit

The report of the Liverpool pilot showed how hard it can be to assess change and improvement. A coding system for audits can help practices assess better the state of their audits and the extent to which the criteria are well formulated and the audit corresponds to the audit cycle. This is explained more fully in Chapter 21.

Audit directories

Practices will always need to learn from each other, not least in setting up audits. Small groups may be an appropriate method, but at the least MAAGs need to publish a directory of simple, problem solving audits (Chapter 14) which have been carried out by different practices, so that practices can contact each other for advice. Or the MAAG could hold a library of such audits as examples for practices to use or adapt.

Comparative audit

Practices are always keen to compare their performance with others. So long as the pitfalls of interpretation are appreciated—such as the dangers of complacency when a practice finds itself to be 'average', and the uncertainty of interpretation if it is found to be in the tail of the distribution—then such comparisons can provide a great stimulus to practice discussions and self-criticism. This is a service that MAAGs can undertake, either by offering central analysis or by setting up practices in groups.

In order to make comparisons between practices, the practices need to agree to assess common criteria to make such comparison meaningful. MAAGs can help by offering criteria lists against which practices can collect data, and then the data can be compared centrally (see diabetes, p. 126). For practices using the same computers, computer templates can be supplied to allow identical searches within different practices (see p. 67).

It must not be forgotten that these data are collected in the course of routine work, on an audit basis, and not with research project rigour. The dangers of regarding such data as giving a picture of District clinical behaviour are made clear by Professor Metcalfe in Chapter 3. Conclusions may be drawn, but with great circumspection.

Individual projects

A further way in which MAAGs can foster local audit is by the development of individual projects. These may be topics which are not widely undertaken, such as monitoring patients' views, or which maybe produce too few cases to be meaningful in a single practice, such as a study of sudden deaths. The MAAG might develop some protocols and offer them for interested practices to participate. This would give experienced practices a chance to try something new, starting practices an example on which to build further activity, and the MAAG some insight into the health and health care of the District.

Topics for such audits might come from the practices, the MAAG itself, the patients or CHC, or even the FHSA or RHA—but again it is important to stress that MAAG activity should reflect that which is needed to help the education and development of primary care, and the MAAG must be careful not to be driven in inappropriate directions by other authorities.

Education

The development of audit has demonstrated educational need. Many practices are developing educational programmes within the practice, rather than always going to postgraduate centres: such education is convenient, relevant, more likely to produce change, and can involve the whole team. Audit facilitators have been reviewing practices' audits and helping them to develop audit plans. General practitioner tutors are increasingly seeing their roles in visiting practices to develop practice education plans. These roles could gradually be combined, with each practice being associated with a tutor to advise on both audit and education.

The teamwork approach to audit has been emphasized throughout this book, and both Liverpool and Oxford MAAGs have recognized the need to appoint nursing and non-clinical members. MAAGs also have a clear role in developing education for the whole team in the field of audit. Since they increasingly employ full-time nursing and administrative staff, they are in an excellent position to run programmes of staff, and full team, education.

VISION AND REALITY

Audit in primary care could have been developed by a high-powered academic practitioner, or health service manager, safe in an ivory tower, just visible to us if we use a telescope, and signalling back to the rest of us a message about audit. In Liverpool, the Professor of General Practice dropped his semaphore flags and joined the rest of us at base camp (Fig. 20.2). Academic input is as important as long-distance vision—being aware of how far it is possible to go.

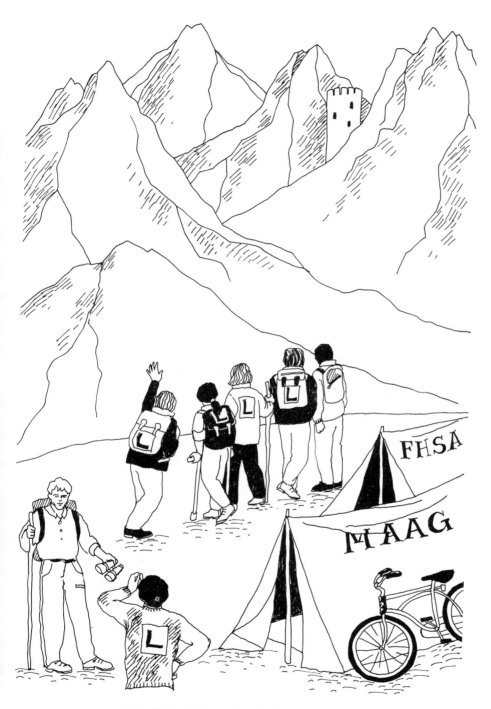

Fig. 20.2 Vision and reality in medical audit.

But we looked around at the whole landscape and saw that there was more than one peak. It is likely that the view from each summit will be equally interesting.

Before setting out it is important to have a secure base camp, and for this it is necessary to have co-operation between management and general practitioners. To begin with, the audit cycle was left in camp, but it is still in full view ready to be wheeled out and used.

More important than anything is the quality of people in the foreground and how they approach the task. They include general practitioners, MAAG members, audit facilitators, an administrative assistant, and an FHSA member. They are close enough to talk without being overheard; they support one another if the going gets steep. Together they ensure that any individual disability does not become a handicap. They are not ashamed to display their learner plates. They appreciate the beauty of the journey, the view from each ridge, and, perhaps most importantly, they never cease to question.

REFERENCES

Department of Health (1989). *General practice in the National Health Service: the 1990 contract*. HMSO, London.

Department of Health (1990). *Medical audit in the family practitioner services*. Health Circular HC(FP) (90)8. Department of Health, London.

Secretaries of State for Health, Wales, Northern Ireland and Scotland. (1987). *Promoting better health. The Government's programme for improving primary health care*. HMSO, London.

Secretaries of State for Health, Wales, Northern Ireland and Scotland. (1989). *Working for patients*. HMSO, London.

21 Auditing audit

Martin Lawrence

Medical audit is an integral part of the medical care carried out by primary health care teams. It has several objectives — to improve patient services, to provide accountability, to stimulate education, to improve morale, and to stimulate research. It consumes resources, both of time and money, and has opportunity costs. As such, it is a topic of care which itself is amenable to audit.

Again, like any other topic of care it can be assessed with regard to structure, process, and outcome; and, as usual, structure is easiest to assess and outcome most difficult. But only if we have some evidence that medical audit produces positive outcomes is it worth reviewing structure and process.

THE OUTCOME OF AUDIT

To demonstrate outcome benefit from audit in primary health care is extremely difficult, for several reasons.

First, and most importantly, audit is not usually conducted on the basis of research rigour, comparing those receiving the intervention with a control group. Therefore, it is always difficult to infer that any improvement derived from the audit and did not occur either by chance or because the group doing audit is a motivated group improving patient care in many other ways.

For example, a survey of preventive procedures in 29 practices undertaken in conjunction with group work was repeated two years later showing significant improvement: but the participants were doctors attending a residential postgraduate course, and so highly motivated to improving practice (Fleming and Lawrence 1983).

To obtain outcome evidence from audits of this type will require research comparing groups subjected to an audit exercise with comparable groups not so exposed. It will be progressively more difficult to undertake such research because audit is increasingly seen not as an 'extra', but as an integral part of care. Practices which are 'better' in various areas of care will have audit integrated into that care, and separating audit out as the cause for improvement will be complicated by many confounding factors.

Secondly, many audits are reported which review patients at high risk or with problems, who then have the risk factors reduced or their problems managed. We know that a repeat audit of patients whose initial results are abnormal will tend to show improvement due to regression to the mean, and audits of this type cannot be offered as evidence of a positive outcome.

For example, in a screening programme at one general practice, 221 patients were found to have raised cholesterol levels as defined by the practice (approximately above 6.5 mmol/l depending on age and sex). A total of 181 patients attended lifestyle intervention, and 121 returned for a cholesterol check at the three months. Of those returning, 64 per cent showed a drop in blood cholesterol levels, and the mean fall was 0.74 mmol/l. The article states that '64 per cent showed a positive response to life style intervention' (Jones *et al.* 1988).

Thirdly, many items of care, for example those related to patients' views, report a very high level of satisfactory outcome even before any behaviour change. This makes any change in outcome hard to detect.

A study of consulting times sought patients' views on consultation lengths of 5 minutes, 7.5 minutes, and 10 minutes. Since 90 per cent of patients stated that they had adequate time to give and receive all necessary information in 5 minutes, it was not possible to show any significant change with lengthening consultation (Morrell *et al.* 1986).

Despite this difficulty it is clearly important that work on assessing patients' views is developed. Not only is patient satisfaction an important outcome in itself, and one which is potentially accessible for the practice to monitor; but meeting the needs of those whom an organization serves is the first principle in raising quality.

Fourthly, many types of audit are not amenable to before and after studies to demonstrate change. In particular, many critical incident studies cannot be reviewed — especially as they may only concern one patient whom it may be too late to help.

Finally, a major objective of audit is to stimulate education and develop morale. Development of audit stimulates team meetings, and even studies which cannot show objective change in patient care often report that those taking part felt the benefit of change (Steven and Douglas 1986; Gau *et al.* 1989). Indeed, one group which failed to show change within their practices concluded that 'audit may only change the auditor' (Anderson *et al.* 1988).

Despite these difficulties, there is some evidence that beneficial outcomes do derive from audit, particularly inasmuch as management strategies of which audit is a component appear to be successful in improving care.

There is evidence in the field of prevention, with feedback of findings followed by improved recording (Fleming and Lawrence 1983; Maitland *et al.* 1991); chronic disease management — hospital diabetics discharged to a systematic care programme were found on review to do as well as those on hospital care (Singh *et al.* 1984); and acute care — wheezy children reduced medication and improved health indicators after their doctors developed a care plan and monitored progress (North of England Study 1991).

In all these cases audit was part of a package of measures to improve care, which included group work by the doctors, development of a management plan, and the review of results.

In improving overall practice performance the system of trainer visiting in the Oxford Region has been widely reported, by which three trainers visit a fourth each four years when re-accreditation is due. Again, this is taking place within a highly structured group agreeing their own target standards for care, and there is a major external sanction (withdrawal of accreditation). But the progress of practices in achieving the target standards set, the subsequent toughening of the criteria and raising of the level of performance expected, and the major educational benefits of the visiting itself are all well demonstrated (Schofield and Hasler 1984).

The need for multiple and persisting interventions to improve the likelihood of change has been shown in hospital audit (Mitchell and Fowkes 1985). It also accords with much modern theory of change, and there are clinical analogues. It is increasingly realized that the long-held view of how to stop people smoking (just tell them to and 5 per cent will) is inadequate, and that the most effective methods are those which involve multiple inputs over prolonged time. The same has been shown for alcohol withdrawal. Why should medical staff behave differently from their patients? Improvement is likely to take place best if undertaken at all levels of the organization all the time. Audit is integral with training and education, and cannot be separated from management in its effect on outcome. It would be to advocate regressive behaviour to try to examine whether audit in isolation has an effect.

Indeed, TQM again highlights the dangers of excessively concentrating on the audit of outcome. Fifteen years ago Ashbaugh showed that '95 per cent of deficiencies are due to failure of performance rather than knowledge'. Berwick *et al.* (1992) point out that 'Quality is an effect caused by the *process* of production', and that 'inspection of final results alone offers little knowledge about the underlying causes in the processes that caused those results'; It is clear from their arguments that not only is the audit of process in primary care more feasible than audit of outcome, it is probably more valuable. Once research has demonstrated the process necessary to produce good outcome, then audit must examine all stages of that process in order to ensure that the route to good outcome is efficiently and effectively followed at each stage and by the whole team.

Conclusion

There is good evidence that medical audit contributes to good outcomes, both for patient care and professional education. Without doubt, that benefit is greatest when the audit is an integral part of teamwork, protocol design, and practice education — indeed, when the audit cycle is completed in all its stages, especially planning care and setting target standards. For this reason, it is justifiable to audit the process of audit with confidence that it provides a good proxy for outcome.

INTERMEDIATE OUTCOME

Intermediate outcome is an important concept in primary care. Whereas outcome is often too delayed and too heavily affected by multiple influences to be a feasible element for audit, certain aspects of process have such a major influence on outcome and can be measured sufficiently accurately to be regarded as outcomes in themselves. These elements are termed 'intermediate outcomes'.

For example, whether or not a hypertensive patient's blood pressure has been measured would be regarded as part of process; whether the treated blood pressure is below 90 mmHg is an intermediate outcome. Intermediate outcomes abound in chronic disease management—blood sugar, peak flow, blood anticonvulsant levels, pain, and mobility, are all intermediate outcomes. But they can be defined in all areas of care: in prevention, patients' understanding of dietary advice, or numbers of smokers giving up; in management, the duration of patients' wait for information, or the speed of response to calls for chest pain; in acute care, the extent to which a practice protocol is followed, or the time between presentation and cure of enuresis.

Acknowledgement of the difficulty of auditing outcome in primary care can be a recipe for satisfaction with simply looking at process. Intermediate outcome is a valuable concept in avoiding this. Being more precise, it is a closer indicator to final outcome than a simple process measure, and it enables practices steadily to develop their audit rigour. Many practices will begin by auditing criteria related to process; once that is satisfactory they can raise their target standards by introducing criteria of intermediate outcome. An example of this in relation to diabetes is shown in Chapter 11.

AUDITING THE PROCESS OF AUDIT

It is curious that, while concentrating on auditing the *process* of care, practices only seem to look at the *outcome* and not the process of the audit. Audit is discussed insofar as it reveals the quality of care, or produces change in the practice: but the process of audit whereby this is achieved is largely neglected. Yet the adequacy of the process of audit is strongly related to whether it produces satisfactory outcome. Practices would benefit from a tool for assessment of the audits themselves.

The Oxfordshire MAAG advocated the audit cycle for use in practices. It needed a system to help practices review how well they were using the cycle: and it determined to use the cycle in auditing its own success in improving Oxfordshire audits.

Agreeing criteria

Great care has been taken in this book to argue that audit can only be effective if precise criteria are agreed, so that levels of performance, and hence target standards, can be set. To define these criteria the MAAG first coded the various stages of the audit cycle.

Coding the audit cycle

Code		
I	Choose topic	
II	Set target standards	Criteria identified against which a level of performance can be measured.
III	Observe practice	Data collected, analysed, and presented.
IV	Compare performance with targets	Discussions amongst doctors (IVd), or including other team members (IVt).
V	Implement change and plan care	Changes made as a result of discussions. Written plans for future management.
VI	Cycle repeated	Repeated once (VI), or regularly as part of a practice programme (VIr).

Different levels of audit were then designed according to the number of codes achieved:

Criteria for different levels of audit

Criterion	Satisfied if at least
Full audit	Five of the six codes present
Partial audit	Codes I and III present, plus either II or V
Potential audit	Codes I and III present
Planning audit	Topic chosen and definite intentions for audit
No audit	

Auditing audits

The MAAG was then in a position to audit Oxfordshire practice audits.

Choose the topic

The MAAG decided to begin with a 'bottom up' policy, by assessing practices' current audits and then helping them to improve.

Collect and analyse data

The audit cycle was entered at this point because with no prior information the MAAG was not in a position to set targets. Four audit co-ordinators (general practitioners with two sessions a week each) were appointed, each with responsibility for about 20 practices. Over six months in 1991 they endeavoured to visit every practice, and succeeded in meeting with 80 of the 85. Information about each practice and its past and current audit activity was collected on a semi-structured profile.

The MAAG's information officer then carried out an anlaysis at two levels.

First, audits were analysed for each practice, so the primary health care team members could see which of their audits included the various stages of the audit cycle. As an example, three audits from one practice are detailed:

1. *Topic*:   Patients' views of health checks
   Status: Potential audit
   Codes: I, III, IV

2. *Topic*:   Cardiovascular risk factor reduction
   Status: Full audit
   Codes: I, II, III, IVt, V, VIr

3. *Topic*:   Consultation rates
   Status: Potential audit
   Codes: I, III, IVd, VIr

Secondly, the audits of all Oxfordshire practices visited were analysed to give a measure of audit activity in Oxfordshire. Analysis of all the audits which were being undertaken in Oxfordshire is shown in Fig. 21.1. This concealed the fact that some practices do many and others few or none, so an analysis based on each practice's 'best ' audit was also carried out. These results are shown in the Figs. 21.2 and 21.3, which show the performance for 'best ever' and 'best current' audits.

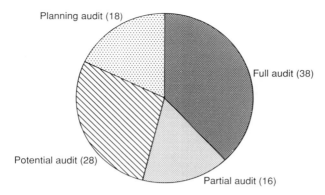

Fig. 21.1 All audits done in Oxfordshire practices, according to level of audit achieved (per cent).

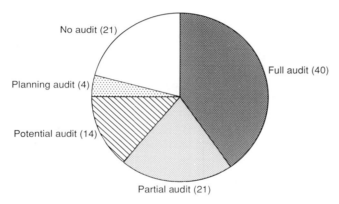

Fig. 21.2 Oxfordshire practices, according to level of best audit which each had ever achieved (per cent).

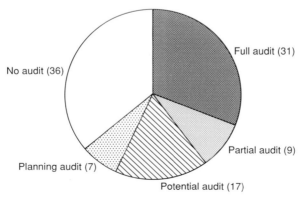

Fig. 21.3 Oxfordshire practices, according to level of best audit which they are currently achieving (per cent).

Evaluate performance

The striking feature of the audits being undertaken at the time of the survey was the number of 'I, III, IV' audits, almost a third of the total (Fig. 21.1). These are audits which involve collecting data, discussing it, and maybe repeating the process; but omit any formal procedure for implementing change, do not include written plans for care, and do not set targets for future performance. The MAAG believed that by highlighting this using the coding system, practices could be motivated to carry out the essential missing steps: in other words, we could point out the deficiency in the *process* of their audits which are likely to lead to inadequate *outcome* in terms of improvement of care.

It was notable that 75 per cent of practices had done some audit in the past, but only 57 per cent were still doing so (Figs 21.2 and 21.3). It is clear that the current level must be less than the historic one (since it is a sub-set), but the reduction was also attributed by co-ordinators to the pressure practices were feeling to complete data collection for the new general practitioner contract, which was squeezing out activity which the MAAG classed as audit. At the time of the review about 40 per cent of practices were conducting audit which included implementing change or setting targets; 25 per cent were conducting 'I, III, IV' audit or making plans, and the remainder were doing and planning no audit at all. The fact that a third of practices were classified as doing 'no audit' in a district where 97 per cent of practices achieve top immunization and cytology targets emphasizes how much data were being collected without evaluation.

Plan care

As a result of this evaluation the MAAG developed a plan to help practices improve their audits.

The practices were divided into three categories. Those doing 'full' or 'partial' audit were mainly being used as a resource to help others. Most energy was directed to those doing 'potential' or 'planning' audit. Regarding those doing no audit at all, contact and encouragement was continued with less expectation of early change.

Setting target standards

Using these criteria for assessment the MAAG aimed:

1. To encourage practices to set themselves the target that every audit carried out will include code V (implementing change and planning care), and where possible code II (agreeing criteria for further assessment).
2. To achieve the following levels of audit in Oxfordshire within nine months: 50 per cent of practices doing 'full' or 'partial' audit; 25 per cent of practices

doing 'potential' audit. Half of the remainder planning. (This target was indeed achieved, with 70 per cent of practices doing 'full' or 'partial' audit, and only 13 per cent doing none, within 9 months.)

Conclusion

There are, of course, other aspects of audit which can be audited besides the extent to which practices' audits complete the cycle. In particular, each stage of the cycle can itself be reviewed — and the practice can examine whether many of the principles outlined in Part II of this book were adhered to. In particular, it is important that audit topics are chosen which cover the whole range of medical and administrative activity, and that members of the health care team are involved, from choosing the topic to setting targets.

The development of a coding system for the audit cycle and the definition of precise criteria for the completeness of audits enabled the MAAG to set target standards for its activity. The MAAG was also able to use the same stimulus in helping individual practices to improve the completeness of their audits, which is the most likely way of producing effective outcome.

REFERENCES

Anderson, C. M., Chambers, S., Clamp, M. *et al.* (1988). Can audit improve patient care? Effects of studying the use of digoxin in general practice. *British Medical Journal*, **297**, 113–14.

Berwick, D. M., Enthoven, A., Bunker, J. P. (1992). Quality management in the NHS: the doctor's role — I. *British Medical Journal*, **304**, 235–9.

Fleming, D. M. and Lawrence, M. S. (1983). The impact of audit on preventive measures. *British Medical Journal*, **287**, 1852–4.

Gau, D., Pryce Jones, M., and Tippins, D. (1989). Satisfactory practice. *Health Services Journal*, **30 November**, 1464–5.

Jones, A., Davies, D. H., Dove, J. R., Collinson, M. A., and Brown, P. M. R. Identification and treatment of risk factors for coronary disease in general practice: a possible screening model. *British Medical Journal*, **296**, 1711–14.

Maitland, J. M., Reid, J., and Taylor, R. J. (1991). Two stage audit of cerebrovascular and coronary heart disease risk factor recording: the effect of case finding and screening programmes. *British Journal of General Practitioners*, **41**, 144–6.

Mitchell, M. W. and Fowkes, F. G. R. (1985). Audit reviewed: does feedback on performance change clinical behaviour? *Journal of the Royal College of Physicians*, **19**, 251–4.

Morrell, D. C., Evans, M. E., Morris, R. W., and Roland, M. O. (1986). The 'five minute' consultation: effect of time constraint on clinical content and patient satisfaction. *British Medical Journal*, **292**, 870–3.

North of England Study of Standards of Performance in General Practice. (1991). Vol. III. *The effects of standard setting and implementing clinical standards*. Centre for Health Services Research, Newcastle upon Tyne.

Schofield, T. P. C. and Hasler, J. C. (1984). Approval of trainers and training practices in the Oxford region. *British Medical Journal*, **299**, 538—40, 612—4, 688—9.

Singh, B. M., Holland, M. R., and Thorn, P. A. (1984). Metabolic control of diabetes in general practice clinics—comparison with a hospital clinic. *British Medical Journal*, **289**, 726—30.

Steven, I. and Douglas, R. (1986). A self contained method of evaluating patient dissatisfaction in general practice. *Family Practice*, **3**, 14—19.

22 Practice reports and profiles

Theo Schofield

A growing number of practices and teams produce an annual report on their activities. Some of these are intended solely for their own consumption, while others are shared with patients or other groups in the health services. Their content varies considerably from practice to practice, but many contain the results of audits that they have conducted and thus can be a focus of audit activity and a means of disseminating its results.

This chapter will discuss the different purposes of practice annual reports and the contribution that they can make to team based audit.

THE PURPOSES OF A PRACTICE REPORT

The purposes of a practice report include providing:

1. A description of the practice and its activities in the previous year.
2. A statement of the objectives of the practice and the extent to which they have been met.
3. An assessment of the needs of the practice population.
4. A plan for services and the use of resources.
5. A contribution to the planning and management of other health services in the district.

Each of these will be considered in turn.

A DESCRIPTION OF THE PRACTICE AND ITS ACTIVITIES

A report can describe the history of a practice team, its current membership, the services it provides, and the significant events which have taken place in the past year. This can make a valuable contribution to the team's sense of identity, increase the team members' awareness of each other's roles and increase patients' understanding of the team and its work. It is very easy to lose sight of all that happens in a practice during a 12 month period and to be unaware of some of the events that have affected members of the team. These can include personal events, such as the birth of new children, as well as projects, publications, or activities outside the practice.

In the past, practices have often been reluctant to advertise or publicize what they are doing. One result is a high level of ignorance about primary health care,

Table 22.1   *Priorities for the practice: The Medical Centre, Shipston-on-Stour*

1. *Patient care*
    We believe that primary medical care includes:
    (a)   Good quality care for patients presenting with problems including:
          accessibility
          continuity of personal care
          competence
    (b)   Good quality care for patients with chronic problems, including:
          diabetes
          asthma
          high blood pressure
          handicap and old age
          psychological illness
    (c)   Comprehensive preventive medicine and health promotion for the whole of the
          practice population including:
          immunization
          child health
          rubella immunity
          antenatal care
          cervical cytology
          family planning
          anti-smoking advice
          education for healthy living

2. *Team support and development*
    The achievement of these priorities depends on the contribution of all members of
    the team, and in many of the tasks the central role is not occupied by the doctors.
    Therefore, developing team working and providing support must be one of our
    central priorities.
        The strengths of each individual team member contribute to the strength of the
    whole. We recognize the importance of personal development and continued
    education.

3. *Performance review*
    We recognize that the process of defining criteria, reviewing performance, and
    modifying practice is an essential tool for achieving good quality care. It also
    develops our accountability, first to our colleagues, but also to our patients and
    society, and if used to reinforce good practice, can have a powerful influence on job
    satisfaction.

4. *Teaching*
    We have accepted the responsibility of being a teaching practice, and this is a
    commitment that we believe should be shared by the whole team.
        It has implications for the sharing of patient care, provision of facilities and time
    for teaching, preparation, and meetings.

5. *Job satisfaction and quality of life*
   We believe that doing a good job is a fundamental part of our quality of life. However, the pressure to provide more and more services of higher and higher quality can impose on the time we have available for home and leisure activities. As a practice we must, therefore, limit ourselves to our priorities and accept that some activities, for example, research, publication, or contributing to the local community, are personal responsibilities.

6. *Financial reward*
   Some of our priorities contribute to the income of the partners, while many others, notably the computer, diminish income. While our standard of living in the practice is part of our overall quality of life we again recognize the need to maintain balance.
   Much of our expenditure is reimbursed in whole or in part, and we may become increasingly accountable for it. Relating our spending to our priorities and reviewing our performance should be part of this exercise.

---

particularly in hospitals, but also in Community Health Councils, Community Units, and even FHSAs.

A relatively small investment in copies of a practice report, made available to patients and sent to other groups with whom the practice relates, can pay considerable dividends in increasing informed discussion and even offers of support.

STATEMENT AND REVIEW OF AIMS AND OBJECTIVES

The production of a practice report is an ideal opportunity to state the aims and objectives of a practice and to review the extent to which these have been achieved. In my own practice we started by agreeing priority areas for our activities (Table 22.1) and acknowledging both their interdependence and the possible conflicts in their achievement. For example, team support, education, and teaching can all contribute to quality of patient care, while the pursuit of leisure and financial reward may cause conflict.

Aims stated in such broad terms need to be translated into more specific objectives as a basis for repeated assessment. Some objectives, for example numbers of patients screened or treated, can be defined fairly easily, while the process of agreeing others can be more difficult and will evolve with time.

Many practice reports are therefore an evolving mixture of description, stated aims, and assessments or audits based on objectives.

ASSESSMENT OF NEEDS IN THE PRACTICE POPULATION

One of the major elements in the recent reforms of the NHS has been to encourage the move from a service in which the providers have chosen what they wish to provide and have been given the resources to do so, to one in which the purchasers define the needs of the population and direct resources appropriately. The same shift can take place in the way in which a primary health care team plans its own services and the way it uses its resources.

The concept of need is often not clear. In the context of the NHS, need has been defined as the ability to benefit from health care (Stephens and Gabday 1991). This definition has the advantage of focusing attention on health gain, and it requires assessment of the effectiveness of many established items of care. This is particularly important in primary care, where many of our interventions have not been properly evaluated.

A broader definition of need is to define goals for health and to measure deficiencies from that goal (Wilkins *et al.* 1991). Assessments based on this approach do not specify health services as a solution for every need. For example, the ability to walk freely without pain can be regarded as a goal, and being confined to the house as indication of need. However, it would not be appropriate to equate this with the need for anti-inflammatory drugs or hip replacement, and a primary care team with strong links with its community would be able to consider a much wider range of approaches to helping a housebound person to overcome that disability. Much of the information required for needs assessment is only available or potentially available in primary health care.

Table 22.2 shows the range of topics and the sources of information that can be brought together by a primary health care team to create a profile of a community and its needs (Schofield and Hipkin, unpublished observations). There are limitations to this approach, particularly the absence of some data, such as occupation, social class, events taking place elsewhere (for example bereavements), and undetected and unmet needs in the population. Small numbers diminish the confidence that can be placed on some items and make comparisons with district based data and from year to year unreliable. However, even a single death from cervical cancer in a woman who has never been screened can concentrate the mind of the whole team on the importance of achieving targets.

Table 22.3 shows some of the problems revealed by this exercise. Some of these, for example housing and transport, are not the direct responsibility of the primary health care team: it was therefore a role of the team to act as an advocate to other organizations. Other issues, for example family planning or termination of pregnancy, could have been seen entirely as a health service problem, but in fact were tackled by the formation of a multi-disciplinary group, including teachers, youth workers, social workers, and parents, in addition to health professionals. In this way a much broader view was taken of the problems of teenage pregnancy and the possible solutions to it.

It is important therefore to include in a community profile not only its problems but also its resources and to identify the sources of leadership in a community and the ways that they can be influenced.

Table 22.2 *A practice profile*

	Topic	Sources of information
(a)	*Population*	
	Population	Practice register
	Population characteristics	Census
	Housing	Local Authorities
	Transport	Local Authorities
	Facilities	Health visitor profile
	Future developments	County plan
(b)	*Health status*	
	Causes of death	Practice register
	Child health	Child health computer
		Health visitor records
	Teenage health	Practice register
		School
	Family planning	Practice register
		District Health Authority Clinics
	Maternity	Midwife
		Health visitor records
	Adult screening	Practice register
	Chronic diseases	Practice register
	Mental health	Practice register
		Community mental health team
	Mental handicap	Mental handicap team
	Chronic disabilities	Social services
	Hospital admissions	Practice register
		Waiting list
	Elderly	Elderly surveillance
		Home care services

Table 22.3 *Problems identified in a profile (Medical Centre, Shipston-on-Stour 1990)*

1. High proportion of elderly people in the population.
2. Lack of housing affordable by young families.
3. No direct bus to local district hospital.
4. A high proportion of elderly patients dying in hospital (including a community hospital) (63 per cent).
5. A low rate of mothers starting to breast feed (59 per cent).
6. A low uptake of family planning services (25 per cent) and a high rate of termination of pregnancy in teenagers (14 per 1000).
7. A high rate of overdoses (2 per 1000) particularly in the 6–24 years age group.

A PLAN FOR SERVICES AND THE USE OF RESOURCES

The next stage in the evolution of the practice report is to pull together the previous strands—a description of the team and its aims, an assessment of the needs of the population, and agreed objectives for care—and to use this to produce a comprehensive team based care plan.

This plan can be divided into separate sections for the management of different patient groups or aspects of the practice organization (Table 22.4). Each topic should be considered under the headings of resources, services, and performance review (Table 22.5): and each topic may well be the responsibility of a subgroup of the practice team.

While subgroups in the practice can look at and report on particular topics, producing an overall plan is a more difficult exercise as it requires teams to examine conflicting priorities and limitations of resources. This can be illustrated by an example from our practice. The group looking after chronic care determined the number of patients in the practice with asthma, hypertension and diabetes and set targets that all patients on regular medication should be reviewed in the nurse-run clinic at least annually.

Table 22.4   *Sections in a team care plan*

Care groups	Practice organization
Health promotion	Patient participation
Chronic care	Reception and access
Child health	Team liaison
Women's health	Drug formulary
Mental health	Computer
Elderly surveillance	Practice report and profile
Teenage health	Community liaison
Terminal care	Multi-disciplinary education

Table 22.5   *Elements in a team care plan*

1. Identification of the target group of patients and their needs to be met.
2. Explicit aims of care.
3. Criteria and targets for quality of care.
4. A plan of care, including the roles and contributions of team members.
5. A plan for the work of the team, including the development of methods of auditing care.
6. Resource implications of these plans.

The womens health group aimed to achieve the practice targets for cervical cytology and also to offer women approaching the menopause a longer appointment with the practice nurse.

The access group monitored waiting times for appointments and found the practice nurses were often booked for more than a week in advance. An audit of their case-load over a month showed that they saw a considerable number of patients at regular intervals with chronic leg ulcers.

The end of the year audit showed that the practice met the cervical smear target, but only 50 per cent of its target for attendance at chronic disease clinics.

This could be seen as a simple issue of shortage of practice nurse time and this may indeed be part of the problem. However, resources are not infinite and other questions that the team may ask include:

1. Are the targets for chronic care review realistic, or can we be more selective in the criteria for referral to the nurse-run clinic?
2. Would increased clerical support ease the pressure on nursing time involved in cervical smears?
3. Would a counsellor or a self-help group be a more appropriate source of support for women with menopausal problems?
4. How effective is our clinical policy for leg ulcers, and should their care be discussed and shared with the community nurses?
5. What are the implications for space, personal time, and finance of increasing the nursing hours in the practice?

An essential part of the planning or resource management process is to define objectives for care, to evaluate their achievement, and revise the objectives in the light of experience. This is the audit cycle in action.

A CONTRIBUTION TO PLANNING AND MANAGEMENT

Primary health care teams cannot make their plans in a vacuum. They will be expected to conform and contribute to the achievement of Health Authority targets and policies, and will be dependent on them for personnel and resources. The strength of primary care in being able to assess and respond to local needs, and in being involved in the development of the local community should be recognized in the planning process. The likelihood of this happening will be greatly increased if teams have data to support their plans.

One of the requirements of the new contract for general practice is to produce an annual report to the FHSA. The areas covered are shown in Table 22.6.

Although these headings are clearly related to policing the contract and received an unfriendly response from the profession, the exercise has encouraged practices to begin to examine their activities and keep data systematically.

Table 22.6   *Information required in annual report for the FHSA*

1. Practice staff
2. Practice premises
3. Referrals
4. Doctors' other commitments
5. Arrangements for patients' comments
6. Prescribing

A major difficulty at the present time is that the collection of data is not standardized, so aggregation of data over the FHSA area or comparisons between practices are very difficult. Some attempts have been made to address this problem (Howarth *et al.* 1989), but there remain major difficulties. A degree of uniformity can be arranged by FHSAs, although this can appear to be imposition: and Professor Metcalfe has already discussed the dangers of interpreting aggregated audit data (p. 28).

There are, nevertheless, major possibilities for practice data to support constructive planning of primary care. Both FHSAs and practices need to work together in partnership to make this exercise valuable.

HOW CAN A PRACTICE REPORT BE PRODUCED?

An important step is to recognize that the process of developing a comprehensive practice report and team care plan is an evolutionary process and will not easily be accomplished at the first attempt. This year's description will raise questions leading to next year's objectives and topics for audit. Collecting data on the practice population and its needs will help the practice develop its plans for future years. Developing methods of audit will enable resources to be allocated more appropriately.

Other crucial steps are to involve the whole team in the production of the report and to identify someone to act as co-ordinator. Initially, a practice report may be the responsibility of the practice manager and a partner, but if it is going to grow and thrive, all members of the team will need to contribute their data and their ideas and in the process become committed to its conclusions.

A well-developed practice information system and a word processor with facilities for tables and graphics are highly desirable. They make the process of putting a report together very much easier and can enhance the appearance of the product considerably (for example, Fig. 22.1). This is especially important if we remember that one of the purposes of producing the report in the first place was to help the team be aware and be proud of their work, and for patients and others to understand what it is that the practice has been trying to achieve.

(a)

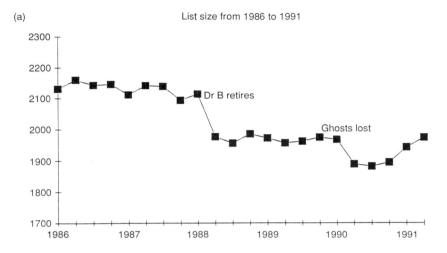

(b) Surgery consultations by age and sex.   Three week sample in Spring 1991.

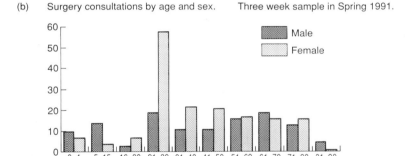

(c)   The breakdown of the mortality figures is as follows:

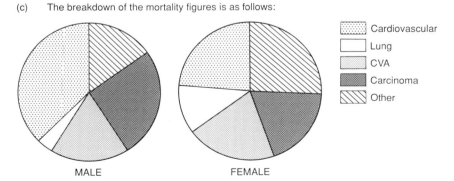

Fig. 22.1 Using graphics to enhance a practice report. (Parts (a) and (b) courtesy of Dr A. Chivers, Jericho Health Centre, Oxford; part (c) courtesy of Dr J.N. Stenhouse & Partners, Faringdon, Oxon.)

CONCLUSION

The practice report is an ideal vehicle for pulling together the audits that have been performed and maintaining the momentum of the audit cycle. It is also an opportunity to review the practice objectives for the past year, and what they should be for the next.

REFERENCES

Stephens, A. and Gabday, J. (1991). Needs assessment needs assessment. *Health Trends*, **23**, 20–3.
Wilkins, D., Hallam, L., and Doggett, M. (1991). *Measurement of need and outcome for primary health care*. Oxford University Press.
Howarth, F. P., Maitland, J. M., and Duffy, P. R. S. (1989). Standardization of core data for practice annual reports: a pilot study. *Journal of the Royal College of General Practitioners*, **39**, 463–6.

Index